ACKNOWLEDGMENTS

None of my accomplishments have been due to my effort alone, nor would they have been worthwhile if I accomplished them alone. I know that this dissertation might have been possible as a lone effort, but it would not be the experience worth celebrating. The most important influences in my life are my parents, Jean and Jim McCawley. My mother and father taught me that I can accomplish anything and they imbued in me the value of education. My life would not be the same without them. My brother and sister, Mary Zinger and Rick McCawley, and their families have also been a great source of support and joy. The admiration from my nieces and nephews gave me an additional incentive to complete this process.

This is an academic endeavor and as such I owe a great debt of thanks to the faculty and staff at the University of Florida. They are too many to name, but a few deserve special mention. I was floundering for a time until my co-chairs, Drs. Barbara Zsembik and Donna Berardo, took me under their wings and gave me a sense of direction. Their mentoring inspired me and helped me maintain my enthusiasm throughout the long process of creating this dissertation. In addition, for their assistance and committee service during my graduate education, I gratefully acknowledge the encouragement of Drs. Leonard Beeghley, Otto von Mering, and Chuck Peek. I appreciate the time they have given to help me become a better scholar. The administrative staff at the Department of Sociology saved me from the grief of bureaucracy, especially Mary Robinson and Sheran Flowers.

I also owe a great debt of gratitude to my support network of dear friends and co-workers. Diana Hannah and Paula Coley persevered in friendship despite my single-minded focus on my academic pursuit. The staff at Fringe Benefit Coordinators, especially Beth Lege and George Zinger, kept the office running in my absence. They gave me peace of mind and a continuing source of income over the past seven years.

My diploma should include the names of my family and friends, the faculty and staff at the University of Florida and F.B.C. who all helped in their own way to make this dissertation a reality. I apologize to those I have not mentioned by name. Know that I gratefully acknowledge your encouragement and support in my graduate career and in the completion of my doctoral dissertation.

TABLE OF CONTENTS

LIST OF TABLES

LIST OF FIGURES

Abstract of Dissertation Presented to the Graduate School
of the University of Florida in Partial Fulfillment of the
Requirements for the Degree of Doctor of Philosophy

SOCIOECONOMIC STATUS AND FUNCTIONAL ABILITY AMONG OLDER ADULTS

By

Dorothy Jean McCawley

December 2000

Chair: Dr. Barbara Zsembik
Major Department: Sociology

With increasing numbers of older adults in the population, research with a focus on healthy recovery among older adults can have an impact on quality of life. Previous research has examined the connection between socioeconomic status and health and found that higher SES and better health are correlated.

This research examines the health-SES link specifically as regards the process of disability in older adults as regards functional limitations, which include difficulty with specific physical actions, which is the focus of this research. The Asset and Health Dynamics Among the Oldest Old survey is a longitudinal data set that includes data about difficulty walking, climbing stairs, lifting 10 pounds, pushing or pulling a large object and picking up a dime from a table. It also includes detailed information about finances and health behaviors. This data set offers the opportunity to analyze the specific functional trajectories of the respondents through the first two waves of data collection.

Net worth proved a better indicator of health function over time than was annual household income. Health behaviors such as exercising, not smoking, controlling weight, and temperate drinking did moderate the relationship between net worth and functional abilities. This group is mostly free of functional limitations, and between 18 – 40% of older adults with functional limitations do recover from the first wave to the second.

CHAPTER 1
HEALTH AMONG OLDER ADULTS

Today the dialogue about aging and the changing expectations of our later years has become an urgent topic. The U.S. Bureau of the Census (1996) has followed the growth in the population of the over age 65 group. In 1994, the over-65 group represented one-eighth of our total population, which is an 11-fold increase from 1990. The Bureau expects another dramatic increase in the number of older adults after 2010 when the Baby Boomers reach age 65.

As we look at the aging process and its theoretical understanding, we see that successful aging may be linked to productivity — no longer a time of disengagement, but of increasing activity. As the number of adults over 65 years of age becomes a larger percentage of our population in the next century this debate becomes increasingly significant. The continuing debate over whether older adults are healthy and capable of recovering if disabled is likely to intensify.

In order to prevent disease and disability (or promote recovery), it is useful to examine how social factors affect the aging process and find ways to facilitate a healthy aging process. We all desire a good quality of life in our later years, which includes high satisfaction, health, material security and happiness (Fry, 1996). The growth in the over-65 portion of the population points to the need to understand the dynamics of health, aging and socioeconomic status (SES), since poor health can undermine the quality of life of older adults.

As we age, our bodies may experience disease, injury or the exacerbation of a congenital condition that results in physical impairment. The "process" of becoming disabled has been described various times in attempts to arrive at some standard model for analyzing the dynamics of disability. Verbrugge and Jette (1994) developed a model that has several steps. First, individuals experience a medical condition that leads to physical impairment, functional limitations, and eventually disability. They called this "the disablement process." Next, they added factors that impact the process, which they label as "risk factors," "extra-individual factors," and "intra-individual factors."

This research uses an expanded version of this model, one that includes health recovery from functional limitations as an alternative outcome to disability. For this study, recovery is defined as a reduction in the difficulty of performing specific functions. Recovery is a significant event when evaluating the process of disability. If we can examine the connections between social factors and health recovery, we can help elders maintain their independence and focus attention to preventing functional limitations, which should reverse the process away from disability.

Studying the incidence of disease is useful for tracking the history of a particular condition. Looking at the functional consequences is more useful for public policy and for the lifestyle of elders and their families. If a disease results in physical impairment, the adult experiences difficulty in performing activities that allow for independent living and self-care (George, 1996). Dependence clearly has a strong negative effect on the quality of life satisfaction of elders, but recovery is possible. Previous studies have demonstrated that recovery from functional disability at some point occurs considerably often (Myers, Juster and Suzman, 1997).

A focus on recovery from functional limitations can help us generate a picture of what resources we need to provide that will allow for continued successful aging of elders today and of successive cohorts of elders. Health recovery is worth study since reversing or delaying the last step in the process to disability means that older adults can maintain their independence longer. Promoting healthy aging contributes to the quality of life and active life expectancy of elders. As Charmaz (1995) notes, recovery is the goal of people with functional limitations. The initial reaction of people faced with chronic illness is to plan to return to their prior level of ability, perhaps even to exceed that level. She acknowledges that sufficient funds allow those who are functionally limited flexibility in their recovery strategies. This research examines the connection between SES and functional limitations in the context of the model of The Disablement Process (Verbrugge and Jette, 1994).

House, Lepkowski, Kinney, Mero, Kessler, and Herzog (1994) note that individuals in the lower SES strata experience greater levels of morbidity than do individuals at higher levels of SES. We can view SES as a risk factor affecting the functional levels of older adults. This has consequences for our public programs that provide for treatment of illness, such as Medicare and Medicaid, and other entitlement programs. As a result, we may realize that investing in prevention, screenings and a focus on healthy aging will be socially beneficial.

Generally, one expects that in the retirement years economic stability is assured through government programs and pension plans in place from previous work history. However, most federal programs are designed to provide a floor of protection and often do not provide coverage in the case of long-term illness (Estes, 1989; Wiener and Illston,

1996). In addition, if an older adult has had a history of poor health that began significantly early in adulthood, he or she may not have had the opportunity to work in an occupation that had fringe benefits such as a pension program. His or her health may have affected the work history, and without consistent employment, older adults may not have a strong pension program, if any.

One comprehensive source of information about the economic and functional status of older adults is the Asset and Health Dynamics Among the Oldest Old (AHEAD) survey. The AHEAD survey provides a longitudinal database for analysis of the relationship between SES and health in the elderly population. The population under study is adults aged 70 and older, despite the title of the survey as "Oldest Old," which is generally considered to refer to individuals 85 and older.

This longitudinal data set offers the opportunity to analyze the specific functional trajectories of the respondents through the first two waves of data collection. Since the data set includes unusually detailed financial information about household income and wealth accumulation, it provides a unique ability to describe and examine the SES/health link among the older adults, the fastest growing portion of our population. Future public policy direction needs such information to guide us into having a healthier aged cohort in the next century.

CHAPTER 2
DETERMINANTS OF FUNCTIONAL STATUS

This chapter includes an overview of the model of functional ability used in this research and of past research relating to the connection between health and socioeconomic status. The focus is on the theory of cumulative advantage and disadvantage. This is followed by a section that covers determinations of SES as well as the role of education in determining SES and health. Next, the moderating effects of health behaviors such as smoking, drinking alcohol, exercise, diet and nutrition, preventive care and social networks are examined. This is followed by a review of literature relating to the covariates. These are age, sex, race/ethnicity, insurance, medical conditions, doctor visits, prescriptions and genetic endowments. The final section of this chapter is a summary and statement of hypotheses.

Introduction

As we pass from one century to another, our population and our experiences present new challenges and opportunities. First we have seen evidence of dramatic increases in our life expectancy, accompanied with the decrease in acute, infectious disease and concomitant increase in chronic, debilitating disease. The result of chronic conditions can be poor physical functioning. Physical functioning, along with adaptation to disease, influences recovery from disease and is also a significant marker for older adults' quality of life. Understanding what social factors are related to the development of poor functional status is informative to gain a full picture of health promotion among older adults. (Guralnick and Lacroix, 1992)

Disability has gained prominence as an area of study because of changes in the health of the population as a whole. For example, at the turn of the last century the medical profession focused on acute, infectious diseases. At the turn of this century chronic diseases have replaced acute conditions as the major cause of death, especially for the elderly (Fried and Wallace, 1992). These conditions, while responsible for death in the over age 65 age group, are also linked to limitations in functional ability, which can be a precursor to disability.

The increasing incidence of chronic conditions leads us to study treatments, not cures (Katz, 1999). Especially when it comes to disabling conditions, we are more interested in increasing the length of time that one is stable or, if possible, the improvement of a condition to avoid total disability. One consequential difference between acute and chronic conditions is that an individual may live for a long time with the limitations of a chronic condition. As Verbrugge and Jette (1994: 1) note, "People mostly live with chronic conditions rather than die from them."

Older adults arrive in their post-retirement years with differing resources, including wealth, health, knowledge, and social networks. The resources that older adults have at this point of their lives are the result of their previous life experiences. Aging is, after all, the accumulation of life experiences and biological changes across an entire life, and a holistic approach recognizes the influences of the past on the present (Wallace, 1992).

Not all older adults arrive at advanced age with disability. Advanced age is not an automatic indicator of functional limitations and resulting disability. Additionally, older adults who do have functional limitations sometimes get better (Manton and Stallard, 1996). Knowing the dynamics of these processes of disability and recovery in community dwelling older adults may help them maintain their independence. A study such as this one also expands our understanding of the link between SES and health by focusing on different health indicators, ones that are closely linked with independent functioning (Wilkinson, 1996).

Arber and Evandrou (1993) point out that independence is perceived on three dimensions. The first is physical independence or being independent in the domestic sphere and being able to maintain one's own physical and personal care. The second is autonomy, which implies the ability for self-direction free from interference. The third aspect of independence is reciprocity or interdependence, which mitigates the negative aspects of help if it is the result of a sense of mutuality. The point of this distinction is that dependence and independence are endpoints of a spectrum and that we reach more acceptable points on this spectrum during the life course. In addition, some loss of independence is palatable if one can maintain a level of autonomy and a sense of receiving that which is owed, rather than offered as "charity." Underlying all this is the ability to function at a level sufficient to maintain self-esteem.

Models of Functional Ability

The combination of an aging population, increases in chronic conditions and life expectancy, and widening economic inequality points to the significance of understanding the mechanisms of functional limitations in old age. If we can clarify the connections between resources and functional ability in older adults, it may be possible to modify social policy to protect older adults.

There are a variety of measures available to determine physical morbidity. Activities of Daily Living (ADLs) focus on activities such as bathing, eating, and toileting. Instrumental Activities of Daily Living (IADLs) measure activities such as shopping, doing laundry, and talking on the telephone. Functional abilities include basic body functions such as walking a short distance, climbing stairs, picking up a dime from a table, lifting 10 pounds, or pushing/pulling an object. ADLs and IADLs are associated with "disability" in Verbrugge and Jette's disablement model (1994). This differs from other schema of disability, including one set forth by Johnson and Wolinsky (1993). Health is a multi-dimensional phenomenon, and as Crimmins (1996) points out, conclusions about trends in disability/functional ability will vary depending on the definition of functional limitations used.

In the Verbrugge and Jette (1994) model, functional limitations occur in the step before disability. The distinction is made that functional limitations reflect difficulty with a specific action, one that is situation-free, and thus not a disability. This differs from other research on disability, which may use measures of functional ability that are context specific. A disability in the Verbrugge and Jette (1994) model is situational and impacts an individual's social role, which is what ADLs and IADLs measure. Thus, this research focuses on measures of function such as the ability to walk several blocks, climb stairs, push or pull a large object, lift 10 pounds, and pick a dime up off a table. These are actions, not activities.

Other definitions of functional limitations include self rated health (poor, fair, good, excellent) or diagnosis by a medical provider. Using the functional limitations listed in the previous paragraph to examine the health – SES connection is useful because they have a direct relation to issues of independence and are less subjective than self-rated health. Another benefit of using functional ability is that it links disease states with environmental influences (Guralnik and Lacroix, 1992). This serves as a valuable tool in describing the needs of the aging population as well as helps in understanding the influences on health status. It also avoids some of the traps of ADL and IADL, which are influenced by socially defined roles and the sociocultural environment (Freedman and Martin, 1998). Functional ability is no less objective than physician's ratings of respondents' health (Markides, Lee, Ray and Black, 1993) and is less subject to complications due to limited access secondary to low SES. This research is focusing on measures relating to physical functioning, especially those early in the disablement process.

The model used in this research to analyze the connection between SES and functional limitations is the model of the disablement process developed by Verbrugge and Jette in 1994 (Figure 1). This model points to the connections between pathological causes of functional limitations as well as the social factors that influence the exacerbation or diminishment of limitations. Disability is a gradual process, and too often we analyze the end result of the serious disability, but not at the impact of activity limitations that affect participation in quality of life (or leisure) activities (Atchley, 1998). This reflects the current thinking of aging as a social pathology (Arber and Ginn, 1991).

One additional "risk factor" that could possibly add to our understanding of the disablement process that is not explicitly included in Verbrugge and Jette's model is the accumulation of resources such as wealth, education, and income. These resources, which determine one's socioeconomic status (SES), are not evenly distributed in our society and previous research has linked SES and health (Deaton and Paxson 1998; Feinstein 1993; Link and Phelan 1995; Nagi 1976; Preston and Taubman 1994). Risk factors are considered pre-disposing because they occur before the disablement process begins.

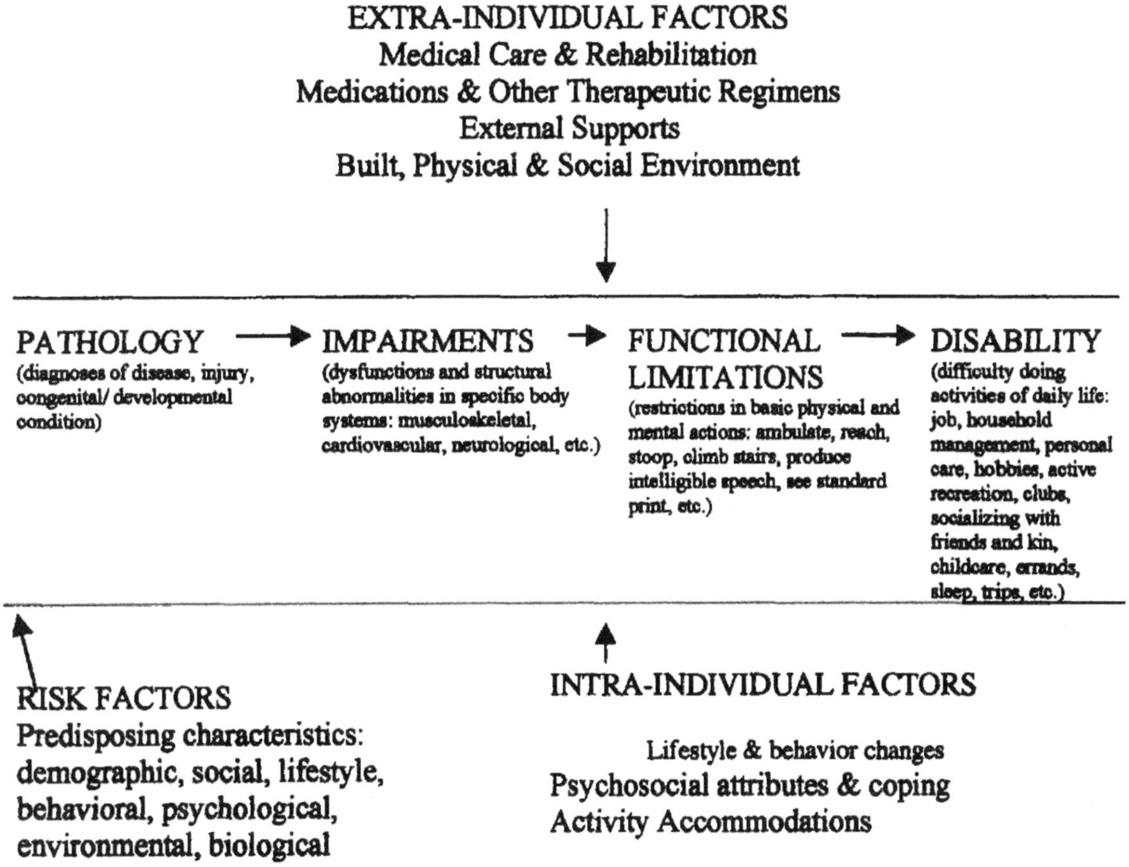

Figure 1. A Model of the Disablement Process (Verbrugge and Jette, 1994)

Socioeconomic Status and Health

Theoretical Implications

Older adults have accumulated advantageous resources in terms of savings, accumulation of a pension, and access to governmental benefits due to the type of employment they enjoyed in their younger years (Evandrou and Falkingham, 1993). Their lack of accumulation may also be the result of disadvantages that they have faced over their life course. As O'Rand and Henretta (1999: 10) point out, "[c]umulative advantage characterizes patterns of divergence or increased inequality over time."

Public programs reduce inequality in later years, but do not result in a total leveling effect among older adults (O'Rand and Henretta, 1999). They cannot counteract the accumulation of pension and wealth over the life course. Individuals with greater income have the option of savings, which, over time, translate into greater wealth. The resulting accumulation can ultimately produce a larger SES-health gap as the cohort ages (Kubzansky, Berkman, Glass, and Seeman, 1998). The theory of cumulative advantage/disadvantage points to consequent disadvantages, such as illness or functional limitations, which can result in increases in inequality at older ages (O'Rand, 1996). In other words, as individuals age, they have opportunities that make it possible for them to accumulate resources. Alternatively, they may face barriers. The more the opportunities, the greater the accumulated resources, the better health older adults will enjoy.

Another consequential aspect of this theory is that, even when negative events occur, the accumulation of advantage may allow individuals with the benefit of resources the ability to recover more quickly than individuals without resources. Aging is not a story of inevitable decline. It is possible for some older adults to reach extreme old age in good health with no functional limitations as well as to recover from health limitations they experience. This research adds to this discussion by providing a description and explanation for elders in the functional limitation stage of the disability process. Disability is one of the most significant risk factors contributing to mortality among older adults (Rogers, 1995). The goal of this research is to examine the relative contribution of resources in the form of finances and in the form of health behaviors/health stock through the mechanism of cumulative advantage/disadvantage theory.

This pattern of cumulative advantage intersects with issues of health and well-being. Individuals who enjoy good health in their middle years have formed a basis for good health in their older years. Individuals who have accumulated disadvantages in their middle years may find their older years even more difficult and as a result experience an increase in inequality over time. O'Rand (1996) outlines the process of cumulative advantage and disadvantage of resources (wealth and health) over the course of one's life that produces stratification of our elders. Initial inequalities in the distribution of resources (economic or health-related) result in barriers to individuals in disadvantaged groups. As a result, over the course of the life cycle, any disruptive social changes result in multiplying the disadvantages one experiences (Uhlenberg and Miner, 1996). Conversely, individuals who have access to resources have access to opportunities to accumulate advantages over the life course. The result is stratification of our elders with inequality in SES and health which may be exacerbated by negative health events.

Mortality and morbidity rates for the upper social classes have dropped in recent decades (Feinstein, 1993) which has resulted in a widening of the health gap between the rich and poor. Elders in the upper social classes may have access to resources that allow for prompt treatment of health and the purchase of goods and services that promote good health and a lifestyle free of violence and negative environmental influences. This gap between rich and poor is also a result of cumulative disadvantage and advantage as we see inequalities increasing with age (Deaton and Paxson, 1998) and for each succeeding cohort of elders (O'Rand, 1996).

Socioeconomic Status – Income and Wealth

Previous research has found a consistent negative correlation between health and socioeconomic status (Arber and Cooper, 1999; Deaton and Paxson, 1998; Feinstein, 1993; Link and Phelan, 1995; Kington and Smith, 1997; Preston and Taubman, 1994; Smith, 1995;), although the exact nature of the causal relationship is unknown

(Cartwright, 1992). One longitudinal study using income found that a period of economic deprivation does predict future functional limitations (Lynch, Kaplan, and Shema, 1997). They did not have information on wealth, and they measured economic deprivation as the number of times individuals were below 200% of the poverty level. The mean age of their study population was about 65 years of age. Income, wealth, and older ages were not the focus of that research. How does SES link to health? Which comes first?

One argument is that poor health limits one's ability to work consistently at better paying jobs, is associated with unhealthy living conditions and limits access to good health care and preventive services (Adler, Boyce, Chesney, Cohen, Folkman, Kahn and Syme, 1994). Smith (1995) points out that ill health also has associated medical expenses that deplete savings and the ability to save. Health in older ages reflects the life history of the individual.

The opposite argument is that living with limited opportunities can result in poorer health. If one has wealth, the household is able to afford access to a preventive lifestyle and better medical care (Smith, 1995), while individuals in limited financial circumstances may engage in less healthful behaviors due to a lack of resources or limited access, or lack of knowledge. Arber and Cooper (1999) found that social class (as measured by last main occupation) was a better predictor of health status than was age, for men and for women. "Access to money, and the desirable attributes that go with it, such as car ownership and the power to buy services as they are needed, depends on life history rather than any special circumstances related to old age" (Wilson, 1993: 63).

Researchers using cross-sectional data to analyze the relationship between SES and health can determine that health and SES are linked, in that individuals with higher

SES have better health (Adler et al., 1994, House 1994). However, cross-sectional studies cannot provide us with information about temporal ordering of SES and health. It is evident that we need to extend prior research to analyze causal inferences between SES and health at older ages (House, Lepkowski, Kinney, Mero, Kessler, and Herzog, 1994).

Some researchers look at the relationship between socioeconomic status and health and assume that we can improve health by adding to individuals' income and wealth (Smith and Kington, 1997). This would work if the assumption about the causal connection is true. Older adults in the AHEAD have a certain "stock" of health that can serve as a baseline for analysis, and with the longitudinal data available this research can examine the direction of the SES effects on health recovery (Smith and Kington, 1977). We can ask, does knowing SES in wave 1 of a longitudinal data set help us predict health status in wave 2? This will not allow for conclusions about the causal association across the lifespan, but does allow for uncovering some of the mechanisms underlying the relationship between health and SES.

In considering the connection between SES and health, it is essential to determine the composition of SES. The AHEAD data set includes information on all possible sources of income for the individual respondent and for the household of the respondent. Another determinant of SES is accumulated wealth.

Wealth, or net worth, includes all assets minus debt, including property ownership, which reflects the "legacy of working life" (Wilson, 1993: 59). Income and net worth are linked, especially for the upper percentiles of the wealthy. The disparity in net worth is explained by looking at differences in income among the wealthier groups (Smith, 1995). Smith (1995) also found that lower income people save less than higher income people regardless of their race or ethnicity, which contributes to their lack of net worth at older ages. In fact, the main source of net worth for the poor and the middle income group is their Social Security benefit (Smith 1995).

Education – Indicator of SES?

Education has been used as one of the factors determining SES. Education, occupation and income tap into different features of SES position (Preston and Taubman, 1994). For older adults, education is stable and so the link between education, as a measure of SES, and health diminishes by age (Beckett, 2000). In addition, education may act in determining health status in other ways rather than directly as an indicator of SES. As such, it may be linked to health behaviors more than SES at older ages.

A good education generally leads to favorable work and living conditions that can have a direct effect of earnings potential and thus higher SES and better health. Education can also indirectly influence health due to the connection between education and better health habits and behaviors (Marmot, 1998). "Educational attainment is associated with the availability of information and with cognitive skills" (Preston and Taubman, 1994, p. 282). As a result, individuals with a good education can obtain information about healthy behaviors and comply with them.

Research by Beckett (2000) found that education and functional impairment are significantly and negatively correlated for individuals over the age of 65. This may reflect the fact that individuals in higher SES brackets and with better education live longer, which may in part be due to behavioral factors related to education as an indicator of self-efficacy. If education continues to hold the same relationship with mortality over time, we can expect longer, healthier lives as better educated cohorts age (Elo and Preston, 1996).

This is what Freedman and Martin (1998) found in their evaluation of functional limitations of adults over the age of 50 evaluated in 1984 and 1993. They noted an increase in educational attainment and a drop in functional limitations over that decade, leading them to conclude that education operates in several ways to improve health. It is associated with a beneficial lifestyle, but it may also be associated with the ability to follow health care treatment plans and to modify the environment, whether that is the physical environment or behaviors.

Manton (1996) also speculates that education gives older adults the motivation they need to stay functional as it also helps them avoid risk factors such as smoking and high-fat diets. The results of his research show that older adults in a low education group were 5.73% more likely to be disabled. Manton's (1996) work was with adults who experienced impairments measured by IADL and ADL, and he found that being a high school graduate makes a difference in disability rates. If disability rates for high school drop-outs were the same as for high school graduates, disability rates would be reduced by thirteen percent.

Education was a measure of healthful behavior by Smith and Kington (1997b) also. They argue that "education may... affect the way individuals can transform inputs into good health" (Smith and Kington, 1997b:108). Greater education gives households access to and awareness of preventive behaviors, avoiding environmental risks, better problem-solving skills, and effective self-care. Reynolds and Ross (1998) found that education has power in predicting good health other than as a credential or that it leads to high status employment. Rather, they found that education is significant, especially if individuals are economically disadvantaged. Other research on older Black adults also found that individuals with more education engaged in health promotion activities

(Ferraro, 1993). In this research, education is used as an indicator of health promoting behavior.

Another view of education that is apart from SES and is an indication of human capital, or the ability to use education to solve a variety of problems, not just as a work-related skill enhancement (Mirowsky, 1998). In this sense, education gives one a sense of control over one's lifestyle, leading to healthful behaviors and fewer functional problems. However, this effect is present only for individuals who enjoy general prosperity. Educated individuals know how to maximize the usefulness of economic resources to reduce any sense of economic hardship (Mirowsky and Ross 1999).

Multiple and Interlocking Mechanisms

Straus (1999, 106) points out that we need to appreciate that "social and cultural forces might be causing or complicating the patient's illness." This is true when we look at the relationship between socioeconomic status and health in the elderly. Parental income has an effect on children's access to education, which shapes employment and earning history. Mirowsky and Hu (1996) found that education was linked to physical impairment. They theorized that a lack of education is related to low income and as a result individuals experience increased risk of physical impairment because they cannot meet their basic physical need for food, clothing, shelter and care. Consequently their limitations prevent them from improving their economic condition which results in concentrating their economic hardship. Mirowsky and Hu (1996, 1091) found "a web of reinforcing effects" in that lack of income, poor health, and lack of exercise work together to compound problems over time.

Life span accumulations of resources may increase the differential between classes experiencing chronic illness. Material resources include current annual income from various sources for respondents and their spouses. Past employment history has an effect on current levels of income and asset accumulation, and health shocks during employment could adversely and cumulatively result in greater inequalities in older ages (Deaton and Paxson, 1994).

Few individuals over the age of 70 are employed, but they have income from public sources, such as Social Security, and from pension plans. In addition to current income, material resources include assets such as home ownership and savings. Older adults who were at a disadvantage during their work life and who suffered illness start their retirement with fewer resources than those who have accumulated advantages. Smith (1997) found, in his study using the AHEAD data set, that net worth is very concentrated in this sample of elders, much more so than is income. Half the population owns 99% of the net worth and the other half has the remaining 1%. The concentration of net worth seems to be among families who are White. The average minority (Black or Latino) household has no financial wealth at all.

The Moderating Effect of Health Behaviors and Health Indicators

Health Behaviors

Verbrugge and Jette's (1994) model of the disablement process points to the existence of lifestyle and behavior factors that moderate the course of functional limitations. They point out that wealth can allow for access to sources of information or services that can alter the impact of medical conditions. Material resources make it possible for the individual to purchase goods and services that can increase the odds of remaining healthy. This includes more than purchasing health care services. For example, owning an automobile allows for freedom of movement to take advantage of preventive medical services or health-related activities such as health club or a jogging park. Wealth is also connected to behavioral factors such as smoking, lifestyle and exposure to violence (Feinstein, 1993). In this way, SES is linked to behavioral factors that can also determine morbidity.

Individual responsibility for health, especially in the face of increasing incidence of chronic disease, can make the difference between functional independence and disability. Mechanic (1995) points out that as chronic disease problems increase in the aging population, the mainstream medical diagnostic disease model is inadequate to address the needs of disabled elderly. Their own intervention and assertiveness to engage in healthful behaviors may be the best source of prevention and recovery. As a result, the wealthier older adults may enjoy higher functional status and be able to recover quicker from limitations.

The quality of health goods and services such as access to providers of care and information about healthy behaviors are usually positively related to price. Generally better quality care costs more, and so individuals with greater economic resources can afford to purchase better quality "health." According to Feinstein (1993) researchers have not reached a consensus about the relative contribution of SES and behavior to health. This may be because SES and health behaviors are interrelated and that behavior is a mediating factor between SES and health, although probably not as significant a contributor as accumulated net worth and income (Wilkinson, 1996).

Individuals in higher SES levels may be able to recover from functional limitations faster because they avoid risky health behaviors such as smoking, drinking and eating less healthful foods. These individuals have access to educational information that helps form their health behaviors. House et al. (1994) note that individuals in higher SES levels are approaching the ideal in aging — experiencing their older years free of significant morbidity and functional limitations until the very last years of life. In addition, they can avoid the stress of economic deprivation that influences the incidence of health problems.

Smoking. Adler et al. (1994) note the strong link between SES components of income, occupation, and education with smoking behavior. The connection is meaningful due to the strong negative effect that smoking has on health. Wilkinson (1996) has noted that smoking has become an identifier for socioeconomic stress. Smoking is closely linked to cancer and cardiovascular disease, medical conditions that can cause functional limitations or adversely affect recovery efforts from functional limitations.

Smoking behavior varies by race and education. Higher educated men and women smoke less than do individuals who do not have a college degree (Berkman and Mullen, 1997). Cessation rates are also higher for individuals with more education. Berkman and Mullen (1997) also note that Black men are more likely to smoke than are White men, but the opposite is true for women. Smoking is an indicator of risk-taking behavior and of public health concern in light of its connection to chronic conditions and subsequent functional limitations (Clark, Callahan, Mungai, Wolinsky, 1996).

Traditionally Mexican-Americans and Puerto Ricans have had lower rates of smoking, but that rate has increased among males in the 1990s (Markides, Rudkin, Angel, and Espino, 1997). Cuban-American males have the highest rate of smoking. As a result, minority individuals (especially men) who are also poorer may have higher incidences of chronic conditions relating to smoking and subsequent limitations.

Alcohol Use. Alcohol consumption follows the opposite pattern as smoking, with individuals in the higher SES levels drinking more than individuals at lower levels (Adler et al., 1994). Excessive alcohol consumption has negative consequences on health, resulting in cirrhosis of the liver (Stoller, 1994). It can also exacerbate other medical conditions, such as ulcers, respiratory disease, and heart conditions, and interact with prescription medications (Council on Scientific Affairs, 1996). Alcohol is also associated with a higher incidence of hip fractures. Not only does alcohol impair balance, but heavier drinkers do not eat a balanced diet and are found to have a lower bone density (Council on Scientific Affairs, 1996).

Previous research on elderly Danes found a U-shaped relation between alcohol consumption and mortality. Both abstaining adults and heavy drinkers had a higher risk of mortality than do light drinkers (Gronbaek, Deis, Becher, Hein, Schnohr, Jensen, Borch, and Sorensen, 1998). The results of this study were the same for older adults as for middle-aged adults and the mortality risk for women was 1.29 for abstaining women as compared to light drinkers and 1.22 for abstaining men as compared to light drinkers. These researchers concluded that light alcohol intake is associated with a lower mortality than is abstaining or heavy drinking. The difference is the result of higher risk of mortality from cardiovascular disease among abstaining adults. Light drinkers have higher high-density lipoprotein (HDL cholesterol) and lower platelet aggregation resulting in better cardiovascular health and lower mortality.

The Council on Scientific Affairs found similar patterns in research of older U.S. adults (1996). Drinking behavior can be damaging to elders' health at any level if it interacts with medications or if the individual is a smoker or has hypertension (Moore, Morton, Beck, Hays, Oishi, Partridge, Genovese and Fink, 1999). Thus, alcohol consumption is a critical variable to consider in an overall view of the health of older adults.

Exercise. Physical activities are no longer integral to work or commuting and are now part of our leisure activity. As a result, lack of regular physical activity has become a health issue. Individuals who do not exercise suffer from loss of muscle mass and are more susceptible to functional limitations. In addition to the direct effect that exercise has in enhancing our health, it also has an indirect effect in that individuals who do not exercise often suffer from obesity (Adler et al., 1994). Ruchlin and Lachs (1999) found that less than half of older adults walk (the most popular exercise of this age group) and when they did walk, most spent less than 15 minutes per walk. Individuals with higher SES and more education exercise more than do individuals at lower SES (Mirowsky and Hu, 1996; Ruchlin and Lachs, 1999) and the older an individual becomes, the less he or she exercises (Bennett and Morgan, 1993). SES and education are indicators of lifestyle, one that includes regular exercise, and helps hinder the development of functional limitations. Exercise is seen as part of a high-status lifestyle and is reinforced by the availability of economic resources in reducing the incidence of functional limitations.

These behavioral characteristics have an effect on an individual's health in a cumulative fashion over the course of the life span. Individuals who participate in regular exercise are less likely to suffer functional impairments, and thus are able to pursue employment on a regular basis and accumulate resources to maintain good health. Exercise can benefit older adults even if they do not exercise when they are younger. Research has shown that exercise, even started after age 70, can reduce physical decline and enhance functional abilities (Cress, Buchner, Questad, Esselman, deLateur, and Schwartz, 1999). Older adults who exercise with weights to increase their endurance see increases in their muscle strength as well as their aerobic capacity. Consequently, these adults move more quickly and are able to carry more weight. Their physiologic reserve is improved, and this helps maintain an independent lifestyle free of functional limitations.

Diet and Nutrition. Additional measures relating lifestyle to health and SES include waist-to-hip ratios and body-mass index measures. The waist-to-hip ratio is a measure of where an individual carries body fat. It can be around the waist, an "apple shape," or around the hips, a "pear shape." The more weight carried around the waist the greater the risk of cardiovascular disease because it indicates a higher concentration of body fat around the heart with resulting atherosclerosis of the blood vessels.

Body-mass index (BMI) is a measure related to waist-to-hip ratio. The BMI is determined by converting height and weight to metric measures and dividing weight by height squared (McBride, 1992). This is a measure of body fat, and higher results are associated with physical disability (Visser, Harris, Langlois, Hannan, Roubenoff, Felson, Wilson and Kiel, 1998). High body fat is associated with chronic disease and low physical activity. High BMI also indicates an increased physical burden on the body. This burden places a strain on joints and muscles and limits the body's ability to move easily. All of these factors increase the risk of functional limitations.

The risk of mortality also increases with greater BMI but is less of a risk at older ages (Stevens, Cai, Pamuk, Williamson, Thun, Wood, 1998; Visser et al. 1998). A moderate increase in BMI as one ages may provide physical resources in the event of metabolic stress from disease. However, large increases in BMI are correlated with an increased risk of disease, such diabetes, arthritis, hypertension and cardiovascular disease (Clark, Callahan, Mungai, and Wolinsky, 1996).

The risk of cardiovascular disease is linked to social class, in that individuals in the lower SES had worse indicators (Marmot et al. 1998). BMI is also correlated with education, indicating that better educated older adults engage in healthier eating as well as physical activity (Kubzansky et al., 1998; Stoller, 1994). The result is a lower risk of functional limitations at older ages.

Similar to patterns in exercising, diet, the other component of BMI, also reflects social class and education. Upper and lower class individuals all prefer healthy diets, but usually upper class individuals know that low fat and high fiber diets are good for their health (Howarth, 1993). Eating may also be a response to stress. Wilkinson (1996) points out that the poor may eat for comfort and as a source of relaxation. The combination of eating out of stress as well as eating the wrong foods puts individuals in a lower SES at greater risk for health consequences of poor eating habits.

Risk also varies by race and ethnicity. Clark et al. (1996) found that 40% of Black women aged 51 to 61 have a BMI considered to be obese and that 25% of Black men were also in the obese category. Obesity was related to difficulty in physical functioning, a link in the path of disability. For example, about 50% of the women and 30% of the men had arthritis and the same percentage reported taking medication for hypertension. Visser et al. (1998) found BMI more predictive of difficulties with physical functioning than changes in muscle mass. They point to weight loss intervention in an attempt to improve the functional performance of older adults.

We cannot overlook the influence of the "food" culture and social structure in the United States in the connections between social class and obesity. McKinlay (1997) argues that we are surrounded by an increasing corporatization of our diet for profit. We are encouraged to eat processed synthetic foods, not the basic, natural, nutritious foods. As a consequence our health care system must focus on "downstream endeavors;" that is, fixing our health problems after they are manifested in functional limitations (McKinlay,

1997: 520). Efforts at increasing healthy eating at earlier ages could result in a cumulative health advantage for older adults.

Preventive Services. Checkups, immunizations, routine screenings, and preventive care are shown to be health enhancing behaviors (Stoller, 1994). However, the amount and type of preventive care an individual receives is dependent on factors related to SES, specifically insurance coverage and access to medical services (Feinstein, 1993).

Generally, individuals who participate in preventive care have ongoing relationships with their physicians. They visit their doctors regularly and the doctors are familiar with their health status. As a result, medical conditions may be detected at an earlier stage and treated more effectively before they become serious. Feinstein (1993) notes that individuals from lower SES admitted through emergency rooms are usually sicker than those from higher SES are. This may be the result of poor quality, intermittent health care received by individuals in lower SES. They may wait to receive care until after the condition is more serious because they do not have a regular provider of care.

Another limitation of U.S. preventive care programs is their focus exclusively on individual behavior. It is a "blaming the victim" type of approach in its underlying ideology (McKinlay, 1997: 529). All this is linked to social structural issues such as moral uniformity that may stem from Puritan roots and are reflected in middle-class values. The medical establishment operates as an instrument of social control condemning certain behaviors and encouraging conformity to other behaviors without considering social context and the wider cultural values. For example, McKinlay (1997) points to the health goal of relaxing to avoid heart disease while the economic system demands hard working dedicated employees. The resulting expectation of behavior change is unrealistic in light of these conflicting values. Focusing on individual behavior also keeps us from recognizing the cultural and economic influences that encourage unhealthful behavior.

While McKinlay (1997) wants to focus on the beginning point of the process of disability, that is, the point at which we experience influences that increase our risk of illness, this research will focus on the midpoint. This is the point at which at-risk behaviors are identified and intervention used at the individual level to prevent the arrival at the endpoint, or actual disability. With the AHEAD data set we can analyze the midpoint and determine if individuals who engage in preventive behaviors have more success at avoiding functional limitations or even recovering once they occur. Whether or not older adults participate in preventive care gives an indication of preventive health behaviors and their connection with functional ability. The AHEAD provides information about respondents' participation in various health screenings, which will be used in this research to indicate preventive care.

Social Networks. Social relationships have an influence of health and well-being (Berkman, Oxman and Seeman, 1992) as well as functional ability (Harwood, Prince, Mann, and Ebrahim, 1998). Berkman and Mullen (1997) note that supportive social networks can reduce mortality risk and delay institutionalization. Part of the effect is the result of improvement in the quality of life due to social connections. Additional factors include monetary support and assistance with routine tasks. A study of women's health found that membership in clubs and organization is especially significant as a predictor of women's health (Moen, Dempster-McClain and Williams, 1992).

Unfortunately the AHEAD data set does not include information on the size, structure, or perception of social relationships. In this case, the closest proxy is the number of children of the respondent and the presence of a partner. These people can be influential in the event of functional limitations, if the children live at home or nearby (Morris, Sherwood, and Morris, 1996). Knowing only the number of children and marital status does not give any sense of the strength of the network, nor its availability or perceived adequacy.

Moen, Dempster-McClain and Williams (1992) found that number of children had no significant contribution to predictions of duration of health for women, but other measures of social support did have a positive relationship with good health. Individuals in good health tend to accumulate roles as they remain active. So, we would expect older adults with good functional abilities to have more children and a partner who can provide the emotional and physical support for continued good health or recovery in the event of a functional limitation.

Social support can be measured in several ways. The help pattern is a determination of the source and types of help offered in through social networks. Researchers have found variation in financial aid, types of services exchanged, and generational linkages (Wilkinson, 1988). One focus of such research is the pattern of help between daughters and their parents.

In the article by Wilkinson (1988) on mother-daughter bonds, she concludes that the study of the help pattern between mother and daughter is complex and influenced by the social environment, the structure of family life, and the changing roles of women. She call for "a more thorough scrutiny of generational ties encompassed by the 'help pattern'" (Wilkinson, 1988: 189). The AHEAD data set does not allow for this thorough analysis, although such a help pattern could be essential in the recovery from functional limitations.

Another tie that contributes to social networks is the marriage bond. The data set includes marital status and the presence of a partner in the household. The marital status of elderly men and women differ, as a result of women's greater longevity. Only after the age of 85 a small majority (54%) of men are widowed, while most women live alone, due primarily to widowhood, starting in their mid-seventies (Arber and Evandrou, 1993). Thus, marital status may help in determining who among older adults is likely to recover from functional limitations.

The divorced, separated, never married, and widowed have much less than one-half the household net worth of married couples (Smith, 1995). Smith (1995) also found that marriage and savings behavior are positively correlated. However, when measuring marital status and its predictive ability for functional limitations, Arber and Cooper (1999) found no statistical relationship.

Marital status has a strong relationship with mortality, with currently married individuals having lowest death rates (Elo and Preston, 1996), benefiting men slightly more than women. Elo and Preston (1996) suggest that this is because of a selection effect, in that the never-married most likely suffer from some health problems. This research looks at functional ability, but we expect to see a similar relationship due to the selection effect as well. Goldman, Korenman, and Weinstein (1995) researched the connection between marital status and disability and found that there may be a survival effect for older adults, such that the differences in disability by marital status are not as expected. In fact, single women in their study were in better health than the married women were. This may indicate that single women are more likely to recover from functional limitations. Recovery was not included in their study. Their work did not include data on net worth nor all sources of income either, which they note as a weakness of their study. This research will include measures of SES to gain insight into the process of recovery from functional limitations considering marital status as part of a social network. This allows for counting members of a social network, but does not provide measures of its instrumental or emotional nature.

Covariates

Demographic Variables

Gender. Women and minorities face multiple disadvantages as they age. Older women and minorities are two or more times likely to be poor than are white men (Choudhury and Leonesio, 1997). Past racial or gender discrimination puts them in a disadvantaged position regarding pension accumulation. Pensions tend to favor people who have had advantages during their lifetime (Uhlenberg and Miner, 1996).

Women live longer, but have more reported illness than men do (Johnson and Wolinsky, 1994). Women are also more likely to suffer functional limitations than men are as they age (Arber and Cooper, 1999; Daltroy et al. 1999) and are less likely to recover (Beckett, Brock, Lemke, Mendes de Leon, Guralnik, Gillenbaum, Branch, Wetle, and Evans, 1996). "Above age 80, nearly 20% more women than men are functionally disabled" (Arber and Ginn, 1993: 37).

It is difficult to determine the exact mechanisms at work here. It may be that there is a link with SES, which was not accounted for in the research referenced above. This could also be the result of a survivorship curve, that the men who have lived to older ages are stronger and less susceptible to disability. In addition, the older men who are disabled are possibly removed from the community-based population and living in care facilities, while women may be more likely to remain in the community.

Additional factors which leave women particularly vulnerable to health and SES inequalities are marital instability (SES is generally the result of husband's work history), lack of opportunities for consistent employment and lack of pension accumulation (Choudhury and Leonesio, 1997). Again, the intersection of SES and various demographic factors put individuals at greater risk of functional impairment. If women have higher levels of disability and longer life expectancy, then the issue of SES is even more critical since women could be living with longer periods of functional limitations and eventual disability than men do. Issues of recovery from functional limitations may also differ by gender. This research will attempt to gain insight into the health-SES connection for men and women.

Race and Ethnicity. A combination of factors place ethnic minorities at a disadvantage when determining functional status. Issues of SES and health are even more essential for ethnic and racial minorities as their population is expected to increase substantially in the next 50 years (Martin and Soldo, 1997). Biology is not the issue here, rather social and economic circumstances affect race and ethnic groups as social entities (Berkman and Mullen, 1997; Kington and Smith, 1997). Especially at older ages, there is less of a race-based difference in mortality and morbidity; social and economic variables explain more of the differences in death rates (Elo and Preston, 1996) and functional limitations (Kington and Smith, 1997).

Previous studies have found that Puerto Ricans and African-Americans suffer from greater disability and functional limitations when over the age of 60 than non-Hispanic White older adults (Jette, Crawford and Tenestedt, 1996). Older African-Americans are concerned about their health and rate their health as worse than Whites (Ferraro, 1993; Berkman and Mullen, 1997). They also suffer from more functional limitations (women more so than men), even though they do not have a significantly different number of chronic health conditions (Ferraro, 1993). Ferraro's research did not include income and net worth variables, but did include education, which was a significantly negatively correlated with functional limitations.

Just as with any grouping by race and ethnicity, Latinos experience diversity within subgroups (Whitfield and Baker-Thomas 1999). Generally Mexican-Americans, Cubans and Puerto-Ricans experience differences in mortality and morbidity from each other (Markides, Rudkin, Angel, Espino, 1997). Some of the differences are due to location of birth (immigrants versus U.S.-born), but some is due to socioeconomic status.

Differences in education between racial and ethnic groups have a correlation with the differences in health experiences. Older adults who are Black experience worse health and generally have less formal education (Bound, Schoenbaum and Waidmann 1995). If they do have a health problem is it more likely to progress to disability than is a similar health problem for a White older adult (Ferraro and Farmer, 1996). In a longitudinal study using ADLs the researchers found that older Blacks had a health disadvantage when compared to Whites but that considerations of SES mitigated the difference somewhat (Mendes de Leon, Beckett, Fillenbaum, Brock, Branch, Evans, and Berkman, 1997). This research used only three levels of income (low [<$5,000], middle [$5,000 - $10,000], income [>$10,000]) and did not include any measures of net worth.

Unfortunately, there is little consensus about how or why racial and ethnic groups may differ in health due to age or SES as many studies do not examine these relationships (Manton and Stallard, 1997). New data is being generated and this research will add to knowledge about differences in SES, functional ability, and race and ethnicity.

Previous studies using the AHEAD data have found net worth gaps by racial and ethnic groups using household wealth (Smith, 1995). This is similar to the results that Brown (1996) found in that the ratio of median earnings of Black to Whites is .6 to .8. The income gap is significantly less than the net worth gap, which may reflect the accumulation of advantage over the life course of non-Hispanic White older adults. Smith (1995) also found that household net worth was unequally distributed across percentiles of household net worth with the upper 5% holding seven times ($655,000) the net worth of the average household among non-Hispanic White households. Brown (1996) found the ratio of median net worth of Blacks to Whites to be .2 to .3. This research looks at differences in functional ability, however, and race is used as a control variable to avoid confounding findings by SES (Ferraro, 1993). Additionally, this research will explore the effect of health promoting behaviors on functional ability.

Age. The oldest old are especially vulnerable to disabling medical conditions. Poverty rates increase with age, especially for women (Soldo, Hurd, Rodgers, and Wallace, 1997). The oldest old are defined as individuals age 85 or older. For the AHEAD data set, which includes interviews with individuals born 1923 and earlier and age 70 at the time of the interview, the oldest old were born in 1908 or earlier. The oldest old may have outlived their resources or they may be experiencing more ill health as they age. This particular cohort was growing up during the Depression era and may be at additional cumulative disadvantage due to the historical period of their work life, which probably started in 1926 (Soldo et al. 1997).

Studies of older adults find that there is a correlation between age and declining physical function, but some older adults, even at the oldest ages, actually recover from disability (Beckett et al. 1996). This is again a point against the problemitizing of old age and assuming that aging is a process of inevitable decline. Beckett et al. (1996) did find that decline increased with increasing age, but there is variability by individuals. Their study did not include measures of SES or health behaviors, which could explain the variability. The purposes of this research is to address this gap. As a result we may be able to determine how older adults who recover from functional limitations differ from those who do not.

Genetic Influences

Our inherited characteristics are not health behaviors, but they do point to the potential of our heath state, so for this study they are characterized as covariates and grouped with health behaviors. Health status in older ages reflects health at younger ages, even back to fetal status and genetic endowments (Smith and Kington, 1997). Thus, some families are healthier than others with cumulative advantages and disadvantages shared by family members. Genetic endowments promote health recovery as they represent early childhood environments (even fetal environments) and the advantages a good environment can contribute to good health in later years. Good health starts in utero with some families being healthier than others and passing this benefit on to children (Smith and Kington, 1997).

Smith and Kington (1997) used the AHEAD wave 1 data set and found several measures within the data set that could be used as proxy measures for genetic endowments. The data set includes age of death and education level of the respondent's parents, which they used to measure the relative good health of the previous generation. It also includes data on the number of surviving siblings and children. They used this all information to create a proxy for genetic endowment and the promotion of health behaviors. They found evidence of "intergenerational health transmission" in the positive correlation of respondents' functional abilities and parents' age at death (Smith and Kington, 1997, 165). Respondents with higher functional abilities also had parents who lived long, even past the respondents' 70th birthday. Similarly, higher functioning respondents had long-lived siblings, another indication of intergenerational health transmission.

Medical Utilization

Existing Medical Conditions: Co-Morbidities. The first step in the disablement process is the presence of chronic conditions or medical events that can result in impairments and then functional limitations. Changes in our environment have reduced the incidence and prevalence of acute, infectious conditions. Limitations on physical activity can have social consequences with the resulting loss of independence and social interaction. Individuals who maintain an active lifestyle are more likely to maintain good physical functioning and be able to recover from them when they do occur. They will have the physiologic resources to regain good functional status (Clark et al. 1996).

Today chronic conditions are increasingly the cause of health problems. Previous studies found that approximately 40% of adults over the age of 65 report activity limitations due to chronic conditions (Fried and Wallace, 1992). Individuals with functional limitations and co-morbidities are more likely to remain functionally disabled than individuals with no other chronic conditions (Chirikos and Nickel, 1986).

Researchers using data from the Framingham Study (Guccione, Felson, Anderson, Anthony, Zhang, Wilson, Kelly-Hayes, Wolf, Kreger, and Kannel, 1994) found that knee osteoarthritis, heart disease, and stroke were conditions most attributable to functional limitations. They also noted that chronic obstructive pulmonary disease and heart disease made significant associations with functional limitations. In the AHEAD data set, we can control for cancer, diabetes, emphysema, heart condition, stroke and arthritis as well as test connections between SES and functional ability and potential recovery of good functional status.

Insurance Coverage. Medicare coverage is available for almost all adults over the age of 65. The U.S. Census (1996) reports that 99.4% of elderly had continuous coverage between Medicare, Medicaid and military health care. However, such coverage is not distributed equally among elders, leaving some groups at greater risk. For example, Mexican Americans have low levels of health insurance coverage and the coverage they do have is minimal (Angel and Angel, 1996). Additionally, elders in poor health or with functional limitations are less likely to have private health insurance (Wilcox-Gök and Rubin 1994). Without this coverage, older adults may not seek care in a timely fashion when it is possible to treat their medical conditions more effectively and increase the probability of recovery from functional limitations. However, the presence of publicly funded programs is no guarantee of adequate coverage for health care expenses.

Unfortunately publicly funded programs such as Medicare and Medicaid do not cover all health care costs. AARP estimates that the elderly will pay 43% of health care costs out of their own pockets (Crystal, 1996). For some older adults this out of pocket payment represents in excess of 16% of their annual income (Estes, 1989). SES status has a direct effect on the amount and type of coverage that elders can afford. This may affect their efforts to receive preventive care or treat chronic conditions that could result in functional impairment and, thus, lower the odds of recovery.

So, the assumption that the elders of our population will successfully age even in the face of chronic illness or disability since public programs will cover the cost of their treatment may be erroneous. Without the full protection of public programs, individuals must look to their own savings to help defray the expenses associated with treating chronic illness and disability. Yet we know that financial assets are not evenly distributed among the elderly (Crystal, 1996), and neither is public or private insurance (U.S. Bureau of the Census, 1996). There is a direct link between the type of coverage one enjoyed during employment years to the adequacy of coverage in the retirement years, once again pointing to the importance of examining the connections between SES and health (Angel and Angel, 1996).

Medical Services. Contact with medical providers and taking prescription medications are indicators of possible pathology that leads to functional limitations. Previous research has found that previous hospital stays are the biggest predictor of continuing functional limitations (Chikiros and Nickels, 1986). Chikiros and Nickels (1986) research did not include prescription medications as a variable, nor did they include net worth as a SES variable (only income). Research using prescription medications did find a strong statistical correlation between use of medication and lower levels of functioning in older adults (Daltroy, Larson, Eaton, Phillips, Liang, 1999).

Another, subtle, economic factor may be at work here as well. Providers of health care are socialized beings and susceptible to economic incentives and the perceived opportunity cost of continuing disability. The subsequent patient care plan may vary depending on the SES of the patient (Chikiros and Nickels, 1986).

Regular medical services are integral to ensuring good health and recovery from functional imitations, since medical advances have the possibility of slowing or stopping the progress of disease to disability (Crimmins, 1997). With increases in life expectancy, researchers are asking if disability-free years are increasing, thus indicating a "compression of morbidity" (Fries, 1989: 208). The concept of compressing morbidity was re-introduced by Fries (1989) who analyzed the concept using data through the 1980s. He points out that individuals in lower SES are not enjoying the benefits of reduced health risks and that their old age will be more expensive if they suffer more disability over a longer period of time in their later years.

Summary of Socioeconomic Status and Functional Ability in Older Adults

Most older adults enjoy a relatively active life; however, about 14% of older adults have some degree of activity limitation (Jette, 1996). This has a negative effect on the quality of life they enjoy and the independence they are able to maintain. Jette (1996) points out that disability prevention is possible and that recovery is a possible and desirable goal for our elders as they experience longer life expectancy and increasing numbers. At the very least, further decline may be stalled or delayed. Another consideration in determining the possibility of health recovery, as well as delayed deterioration, is understanding the mechanisms that increase or decrease the risk of functional limitations at older ages.

Figure 2 is the conceptual model proposed for this research that incorporates the correlates described above. Education is in the health behavior box. In this research education will serve as an indication of self-efficacy regarding healthy behaviors.

Generally, individuals at lower SES suffer poorer health. They tend to adopt more risky health behaviors (House et al. 1994) and have an accumulation of poor health and a lack of resources such education, income and net worth. As House et al. (1994) point out, the accumulated effect of psychosocial risk factors is harder on the physiology of older adults due to biological declines that occur with age. The stratification that accumulates over the course of a lifetime leaves elders particularly vulnerable.

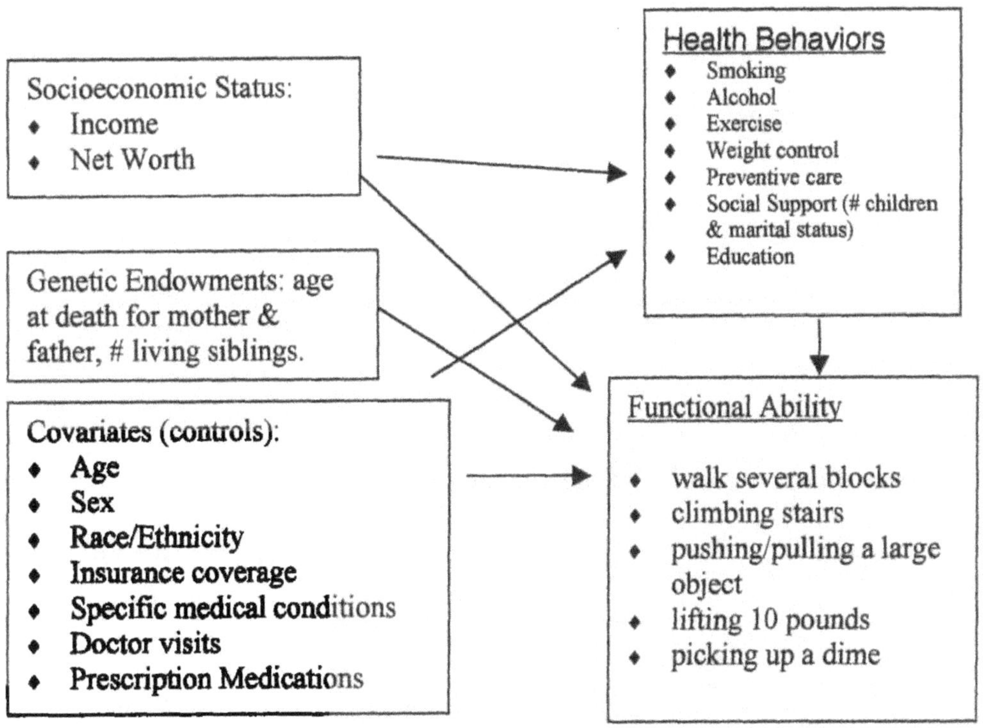

Figure 2. Conceptual Model of the Effects of SES and Health Behaviors on Functional Ability

There is a feedback loop between health and SES, and with cross-sectional data it is difficult to see where the loop begins. Longitudinal data is useful in this endeavor to determine the causal relationship between SES and functional status. Elders are a heterogeneous population with great variation in their functional abilities, and studying change in functional ability over time is a helpful tool in understanding the source of variability and improving the ability to promote health recovery (Jette, 1996).

The disablement process provides a model for examining different outcomes of functional limitations. This model is useful as a basis for determining the relationship of SES and functional status as well as any moderating effects from preventive health behaviors and the relative contribution of income versus net worth to the likelihood of recovery from functional limitations.

Hypotheses

In light of previous research in this area, this research will focus on six hypotheses, as follows:

1) A significant proportion of older adults are free of functional limitations and some of those older adults who do suffer from functional limitation recover from them within two years.

2) Individuals with greater economic resources have stronger functional status.

3) Individuals with greater economic resources are less likely to suffer a decline in their functional status.

4) Individuals with greater economic resources are more likely to recover from functional limitations when they occur.

5) Income and net worth will affect functional limitations differently depending on the functional status of the individual:

   a) Net worth is a better predictor of a stable state regarding functional limitations across both waves of data. Individuals with a higher net worth will be more likely to experience a stable state with no functional limitations, while the opposite is likely to be true for individuals with lower net worth. This is due to the accumulative advantage of a higher net worth or disadvantage of a lower net worth.

b) Income is a better predictor of a transition state regarding functional limitations across both waves of data. Individuals with a higher income will be more likely to recover from functional limitations experienced in wave 1 by wave 2. Individuals with a lower income will be more likely to suffer a decline between Waves. This is due to the current onset of the disabled state and the need for more accessible resources to improve the functional status.

6) Intervening health behaviors will modify the relationship between socioeconomic status and health.

CHAPTER 3
THE SURVEY OF ASSETS AND HEALTH DYNAMICS AMONG THE OLDEST OLD

Research Sample

Data

The Assets and Health Dynamics Among the Oldest Old (AHEAD) survey is a national panel study designed to be used for analysis of older Americans and their experiences with health, finances and families. This is an ongoing longitudinal survey of community based individuals born in 1923 and earlier. The initial sample of 7,447 respondents were taken from the Health and Retirement Survey (HRS) screenings of area probability household sample. Additional respondents aged 80 and older were taken from the Medicare Master Enrollment File (HCFA) for a total of 8,221 respondents. The dual sampling frame was used to test for bias in the selection criteria. Additionally, Mexican-Americans, African-Americans, and Floridians were sampled at 1.8 times the probability as the general population.

The data are organized into three waves with plans to accumulate additional waves of information merged as part of the HRS. Wave 1 includes data that were collected between October 1993 and July 1994 and wave 2 data that was completed in May 1996. The survey was sponsored by the National Institute on Aging. The Institute for Social Research at the University of Michigan oversees the data collection.

The designers of the AHEAD data set recognized the importance of evaluating the interaction of health status and financial well being for setting public policy (Myers,

Juster and Suzman, 1997). As a result they have gathered detailed information at a household level about health, finances and family relationships. This makes the AHEAD an extremely useful data set for determining the direct effect of SES, and its indirect effect through health behaviors, upon the health status of the elders of the United States.

The AHEAD data set is designed to examine the health and economic dynamics of the oldest old. The data set includes detailed information on all sources of household income and net worth, presence or absence of functional status, details of medical diagnoses and health care services, participation in preventive health behaviors as well as limited data on the respondents' parents, siblings, children and grandchildren. This data set makes a unique contribution to research in its richness of detail regarding the health and economic condition that is critical to understanding the SES/health relationship.

An additional benefit of the AHEAD data set is that is it longitudinal. Longitudinal data provide a good picture of onset and desistance of medical conditions that provides us with models of individual health experiences not available with cross-sectional data. With these data researchers can determine the relationship between SES and health for individual cases and categorize respondents by stability or change over time. It is possible to determine the order in which changes occur in functional status and the relationship between functional status, SES and health behaviors among the oldest old. We can then analyze the benefit of knowing SES at wave 1 and functional ability at wave 2 and determine if that knowledge gives us insight into the causative relationship between SES and health over this time period. Through longitudinal data we gain the ability to examine the chronological and developmental course of the relationship between SES and health.

The concepts of "successful aging" and "compression of morbidity" need careful study if we want to encourage them in our rapidly aging society. What social factors influence the continuing good health of the oldest old? Ensuring quality of life for older adults as well as freedom from disability and dependence saves time, money, and emotional distress.

Another advantage of the AHEAD data set and this research is that the functional status will be unbundled into particular activities. Prior research tends to create indices or scales combining various measures of ADL, IADL or functional limitations. Each of these measures of functional ability (walking, climbing, pushing/pulling, lifting and picking up a dime) are influenced by different environmental, social, and physical factors. By analyzing the SES/health connection for each of these independently we eliminate the possibility of complicating upper body versus lower body issues. In this way it is possible to see if the relationship between SES and health varies by specific functional abilities, since different pathologies may influence each of the functional abilities diversely.

The SES/health link is a consequential one to study in this age group for several reasons. First, we will all hopefully be in this category at some point in our lives, and the number of the U.S. population who are aging is increasing. To examine the factors influencing a happy old age aids the oldest old as well as the following generations that are responsible for their care and support. It is informative to see if the SES/health link is the same for the oldest old as it is for other age groups. Secondly, this group is at a unique stage. They have probably accumulated all the net worth and education possible for them, so there is a limit to the question of "reverse causation" (that is, health causing wealth) from this point forward.

The AHEAD data set also offers us information about health behaviors of the oldest old and their impact on functional ability. Does a lower risk lifestyle have an effect on functional ability at older ages? If so, it is not too late for even the oldest old to make changes in health behaviors in order to improve their health status.

This group can also help us recognize the social influences on our health status. They have experienced a lifetime of social forces and influences that have determined their social standing and resulting good or bad health. Critically analyzing this through measures of SES can help succeeding generations to choose a different course.

Sample

The AHEAD wave 1 includes interviews with 8,221 non-institutionalized individuals from 6,047 different households, with a response rate of 80.4% and a dual sampling frame for respondents aged 80 and older. The dual sampling frame, by the HRS and HCFA for the over 80 portion of the sample, was used to eliminate sampling bias. The households surveyed contained at least one individual 70 or older (born prior to 1923) and his or her spouse. Some surveys were conducted face-to-face (especially if the respondent was over age 80), and others took place over the phone depending on the respondent's preferences. The study was designed to over-sample individuals of Black and Hispanic race/ethnicity as well as people living in Florida. Analyses use weighted data unless otherwise indicated.

This study sample will include all individuals who completed the financial, health and behavior sections of the survey in waves 1 and 2. Only survivors are included since this research is trying to determine the influences on transitions in functional ability between waves. The combined sample of wave 1 and wave 2 respondents used in this study is 6,237 individuals. The variables used are summarized in Table 1 on page 49 and the descriptive statistics are summarized in Table 3 on page 58.

One limitation of using this data set is that only three waves of data are available at this time and the waves are only two years apart (this research uses the first two waves). This, however, does allow us a first glimpse at the transitions between functional states among the oldest old, recognizing that recovery from functional limitations may take more time than two years. There is a possibility of the opposite situation as well. With these data we do not know the picture in the intervening time frame. Verbrugge, Reoma and Gruber-Baldini (1994) found that post-hospital older adults improved for a month or two, but then their health declined. They noted that functional ability is variable for the first year following a hospital stay. Respondents could experience functional limitations and recovery several times between waves of data collection.

Other research found that lower body limitations were less likely to resolve than upper body limitations (Wolinsky, Stump, Callahan, and Johnson 1996). Since most of the functional measures in the research are of the lower body, we may have consistency across waves. Any patterns shorter than two years in duration are obscured by the schedule of interviews. As a result, researchers may overestimate the stability of functional status.

Functional status is the third step in the main pathway of Verbrugge and Jette's disablement process model. It is a point in the process where we can observe how physical dysfunctions operate in the lived experiences of the oldest old. This point is also before complete disability, as would be measured by ADLs and IADLs. As such, it is divorced from social definitions and role responsibilities, and any biases this might cause in answers from the respondents. Additionally, it may explain a point in the process before the need for nursing homes or other institutional aids and at which recovery is possible. Jette (1999) called for more longitudinal studies isolating the steps of the disablement process for a more thorough analysis of the critical risk factors at each point in the pathway. This research attempts to do that.

The AHEAD study only peripherally addresses issues of access to health care and barriers to adequate rehabilitation from physical impairments. Respondents are asked about their visits to various providers, but are not asked if they did not see a provider due to access limitations or other barriers to care. The data do not include measures of convalescence nor measures of social networks nor social support. These would be beneficial additions to the study as would questions related to difficulties seeing a provider, whether they are related to transportation issues, cost of care, or lack of availability of providers. The Institute for Social Research has gathered thorough information on the health and wealth status of the respondents.

The data set is also limited by problems common to all longitudinal research, such as attrition due to death and those lost to follow-up. This could be a problem when analyzing health care issues, as individuals more frail may die between waves of data collection. As a result, their experiences are not included in this analysis which may affect our understanding of the trajectory of individuals with greater functional limitations. For the second wave of interviews, 9% of respondents had died between waves, and 11.1% were lost through attrition or did not respond for other unspecified reasons. However, 88.9% of the baseline respondents have provided interviews at all waves in which they were eligible.

Additionally there are problems with confounding cohort effects. Historically, this cohort grew up before we had the medical knowledge we have today which guides our health behaviors. For example, smoking was a popular pastime; cigarettes were passed out on airplane flights. Today, we know the detrimental effects of cigarette smoking and we cannot know what health behaviors we would have seen among this cohort if they had the knowledge we have today. In addition, they lived through a time of segregated school and health care systems. As a result, it is difficult to know if the study results will be applicable to this cohort only or generalizable to the older population of succeeding cohorts or if patterns observed are typical or normative aging. Other measurement limitations will be addressed specifically for each set of variables.

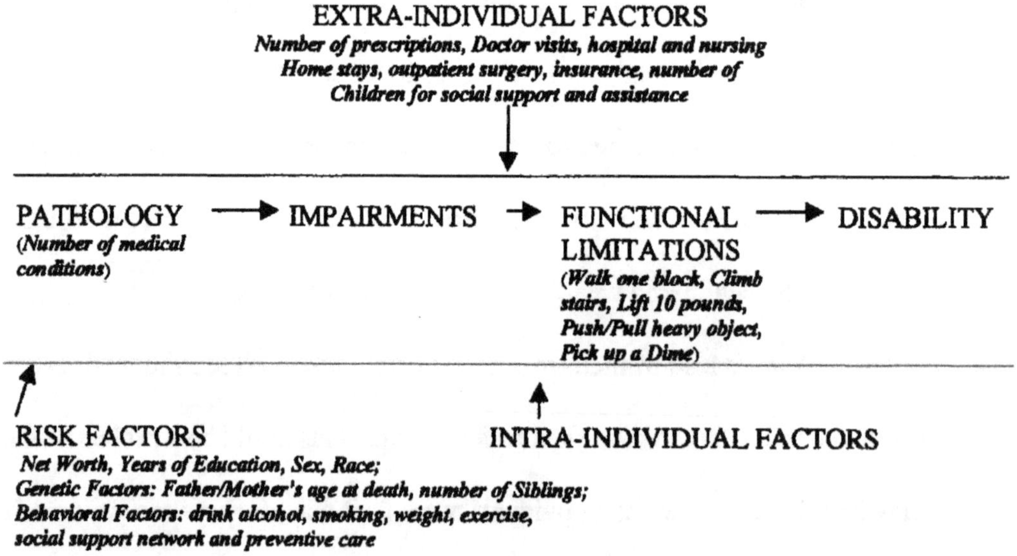

Figure 3. Modification of the Model of the Disablement Process (Verbrugge and Jette, 1994) Showing Variables used in this Research

Measures

The data from Waves 1 and 2 of the Assets and Health Dynamics Among the Oldest Old (AHEAD) were used to analyze the relationship between socioeconomic status (SES) and functional limitations. The wording for selected questions from the AHEAD codebook is included in Appendix A. The model presented by Verbrugge and Jette (1994) is used as the basis for the design of the study. Variables are shown in Table 1.

Functional Performance

The response variable is functional performance. The functional performance indicators in both waves are: walking several blocks, climbing one flight of stairs, pushing or pulling large objects, lifting weights over 10 pounds, and picking up a dime from the table. Respondents were eliminated if they said they "Don't do" the activity, but not because of health reasons. The individuals may not have the occasion to perform these activities, such as not being around stairs, for example. As a result, the response does not provide meaningful information on physical ability, just on environmental limitations and opportunities (Guralnik and Lacroix, 1992). Using functional performance to measure health status has several advantages. In this research, each measure is modeled separately. Aggregating the scales in a meaningful fashion is difficult and may mask difficulties with specific tasks and therefore underestimate the exact level of difficulty with functioning (Guralnik and Lacroix, 1992).

Measures of functional performance have advantages over basing measures of health on medical diagnoses because the existence of a medical diagnosis may be compromised by access to care issues, which are related to SES. Analyzing improvements in functional ability allows for a description of the elders who avoid moving into complete disability.

Table 1. Variable Description and Coding

Variable	Description
Functional Performance (0=no difficulty, 1=difficulty)	
Walking [a,b]	difficulty walking several blocks
Climbing [a,b]	difficulty climbing one flight of stairs
Pushing/ Pulling [a,b]	difficulty pushing/pulling a large object
Lifting [a,b]	difficulty lifting 10 pounds
Pick up a Dime [a,b]	difficulty picking up a dime off a table
Socioeconomic Status	
Income[a]	Total annual household income
Net Worth[a]	All assets minus all debts, including any debt for mortgage in total dollar amount
Health Behaviors	
Smoking[a]	Never smoked, former smoker, current smoker
Alcohol Use[a]	0=abstainer; Light drinker=1-2 drinks; Drinker=3+ drinks/day
Exercise[b]	Vigorous activity three times a week over the past 12 months 0=non exerciser 1=exerciser
Body Mass Index[a]	Weight & Height ratio: Underweight (BMI <18.5); Normal weight (BMI between 18.5 and 24.9); Overweight (BMI >24.9)
Screenings[b]	Number of health care screenings for breast cancer, prostate cancer, cholesterol, cervical cancer, or had a flu shot or breast self-exam: Women: 3* the number of screenings; Men: 5*the number of screenings.
Social networks[a]	Number of children ever had Marital Status: 0=no partner; 1=married or co-habiting
Education[a]	Years of education completed
Covariates	
Genetic Endowments	
Mother's age[a]	Mother's age if living. If deceased, her age at death
Father's age[a]	Father's age if living. If deceased, his age at death
Siblings[a]	Number of siblings still alive
Sex[a]	Sex: 0=male; 1=female
Age[a]	Age at interview
Race[a]	Race/ethnicity: Non-Latino White, African-American, or Other (Latino, Asian, or Native American)
Medical Conditions[a]	Total number present of the following: cancer, diabetes, emphysema, heart condition, stroke, or arthritis
Health Insurance[a]	Three variables: 1) Medicaid = presence or absence of Medicaid, 2) Government Insurance = other Government sponsored ins (Medicare Part A, CHAMPUS), or 3) private pay insurance = Medicare supplements or individual coverage.
Doctor Visit[a]	Respondent visited a doctor in the past 12 months 0=no visits; 1= at least one visit
Prescriptions[a]	Number of prescription medications taken each month

Source: AHEAD

a Wave 1

b Wave 2

Studies have shown that these functional limitations are correlated with many measures of health, such as self-reported health, work disability, IADLs, and ADLs (Johnson and Wolinsky 1993; Waldron and Jacobs 1988). This measure is less subjective than self-reported health, which is useful because it provides a specific level of performance for comparison. It is easily observable to the respondent, compared to some medical conditions, but has not progressed into disability, can be treated to maintain community independence with less costly medical care.

The measures of functional performance include upper and lower body. Walking, and climbing focus on the lower body and its functioning, while lifting 10 pounds and pushing/pulling a heavy object is a measure of both upper and lower body, and picking up a dime is upper body performance. Difficulty with any of these activities can lead to a reduction in ADL or IADL performance. For example, if lifting is a problem, that could reflect problems with reaching, which could mean the individual would eventually be unable to dress or perhaps to grocery shop and unload groceries in the home.

For this research, we focus on the change in functional performance from wave 1 to wave 2. If an individual reports no problem with the measure of functional performance in waves 1 and 2, then the variable is coded as stable with no limitations. If a respondent has difficulty in waves 1 and 2, then the variable is coded as stable, limitations. If an individual has difficulty in wave 1, but is recovered by wave 2, then the variable is coded as recovered. If the respondent had no difficulty in wave 1, but difficulty in wave 2 the variable is coded as declined.

Approximately one-third of respondents in wave 1 experienced some level of difficulty with the functional performance measures, except the ability to pick up a dime from a table (see Table 3). The most difficulty was experienced with walking several blocks (37.5%) and pushing or pulling heavy objects (36.7%). The least difficulty was experienced with picking up a dime from a table (8.3%). In wave 2 all measures increased in the percentage of respondents reporting some level of difficulty with the functional performance measures. Again, the most difficulty was reported with walking several blocks (45.2%) and the least with picking up a dime (11.5%). The second most reportedly difficult task was pushing or pulling a large object followed by lifting 10 pounds and finally climbing one flight of stairs.

Socioeconomic Status

Independent variables will include income and net worth for each household and the educational level of older adults, all measured in wave 1. The mean household income for the respondents in wave 1 was $25,191.94 and ranged from $0.00 to $700,000. For this research income is divided into deciles as shown in Table 2. Household income is measured with a variable constructed by AHEAD staff summing across all household members the amount of income from the following sources:

- Social Security
- Supplemental Security
- Welfare
- Veterans' benefits
- Rental income
- Business
- Farm
- IRA
- Annuity income
- Retirement pension income
- Stock income
- Income from bonds
- Income from dividends or interest on savings or checking accounts or CDs, bonds or treasury bills
- Income from work (including self-employment)
- Any other sources of income.

Net worth includes all other forms of economic resources measured as the total dollar value of all assets owned by household members minus any debts, including the mortgage. This is also a derived variable using assets such as:

- The value of real estate holdings
- Business holdings
- IRA holdings
- Retirement pensions
- Stock ownership
- Mutual fund ownership
- Checking and savings accounts
- Treasury bills and certificates of deposit
- Savings bonds
- Ownership of means of transportation
- Value of jewelry and collections
- Debts owed to respondent
- Rights in a trust or estate

Debts were subtracted from assets to derive the variable for net worth.

- Mortgage
- Utilities
- Credit card balances
- Medical debts
- Life insurance policy loans
- Loans from relatives
- Real estate tax
- Home insurance

Net worth was measured as a total of all assets minus all debt, including home mortgages. Net worth had a larger range and mean than household income. The mean net worth was $182,765 and it ranged from -$285,000 to $14,655,000. Both income and net worth were divided into deciles for regression analysis (Table 2).

Health Behaviors

The AHEAD data set includes information on preventive care behaviors that affect health. The data for smoking, drinking, and BMI are used from wave 1 to establish a baseline. Also, the questions were changed for wave 2 and did not include useful information, such as status as a former smoker. Wave 2 questions included exercise activity and participation in health screenings, which were not asked in wave 1.

Table 2. Decile Ranges for Income and Net Worth

Decile	Income Range	Net Worth Range
1	$0 – 5,900	-$285,000 - +$570
2	6,000 – 8,976	600 – 13,200
3	9,000 - 11,988	13,500 – 35,700
4	12,000 – 14,940	35,712 – 59,200
5	14,976 – 17,820	59,500 – 86,200
6	18,000 – 21,842	86,500 – 120,900
7	22,000 – 26,960	121,000 – 167,000
8	27,000 – 33,600	167,900 – 247,000
9	34,000 – 47,600	247,500 – 422,500
10	48,000 – 700,000	423,000 – 14,655,000

The first health behavior is smoking. Respondents are coded into 1 of 3 categories: 1) non-smoker at wave 1, 2) former smoker at wave 1, and 3) current smoker at wave 1. The referent category is non-smoker.

Another health behavior is alcohol consumption. Details about alcohol consumption include the number of drinks per day. Respondents were coded according to the number of drinks consumed each day. This resulted in three categories: 1) abstains from alcohol (0 drinks per day), 2) light drinker (2 or less drinks per day), and 3) drinker (3+ drinks per day). The referent category is abstaining.

Respondents were also asked about their participation in vigorous activity in wave 2, but the question was not included in wave 1. The question covers physical activity including sports, heavy housework, or a job that requires physical labor. Respondents were asked whether they participated in physical activity three times a week or more over the past 12 months.

An additional behavioral variable related to nutritional status and physical activity is the imputed body mass index based on the height and weight of the respondents at both waves. The following categories of body size were used: 1) underweight (BMI less than 18.5), 2) normal weight (BMI between 18.5 and 24.9), or 3) overweight (BMI over 24.9). The referent category is normal weight.

The respondents were asked about preventive care services in wave 2, but not in wave 1. They were asked if they had completed or received any of the following: a) flu shot, b) blood test for cholesterol, c) self-test for breast cancer, d) mammogram, e) pap smear, and f) prostate cancer screen since wave 1? Items a, b, c, d, and e will be included for women. Items a, b, and f will be included for men. For each test completed, men will receive 5 points and women will receive 3 points. The scoring calibrates a single scale. The preventive care scale will range from 0 (no screens completed) to 15 (all screens completed).

Education is measured as the number of years of formal schooling the respondents had, with a maximum of 17+ years. The mean number of years of schooling is 10.8 with a range of 0 (1.7%) to 17+ (5.6%) years. Approximately 11% of the respondents completed eighth grade and 30% of the group completed high school and 27% had some college or graduated from college.

The final measure used in this section is of social networks. Unfortunately neither wave includes any information about social networks nor social support. The closest proxy for this is the number of children, assuming that they interact with the respondents, and marital status. The data used is number of children and presence of a partner.

Overall this group follows healthy behaviors, except for weight control. Only 9.7% of the respondents are current smokers with 48.2% never smoking and 42% quitting before wave 1. Eighty-nine point two percent of the group abstains from alcohol or consumes less than one alcoholic drink per day. Slightly less than one-third of the respondents (29.3%), however, engaged in regular vigorous exercise. This could explain the 44% of the respondents who remained overweight between Waves 1 and 2, with a BMI over 24.9. Two point seven percent remained underweight and 11% lost weight while nearly 5% gained weight. The remaining 38% maintained a BMI between 18.5 and 24.9, which is an appropriate weight for their height.

The AHEAD respondents indicated if they participated in preventive care, which included screenings for cholesterol, prostate cancer, breast cancer, cervical cancer, receiving a flu shot, or performing a breast self-exam. The mean score for preventive screens was 9.47 overall. Men received an average score of 10.8, but because the value applied to each screening was 5 points, this means they obtained approximately 2.2 screenings of the total 3 available (cholesterol, flu, prostate). The average score for the women of 8.6, divided by the score per screening of 3, results in a slightly higher participation in preventive screenings of 2.9 of the total 5 available (flu, cholesterol, pap smear, breast self-exam, mammogram). The most popular screening for men was prostate screen (47.5% of the men receiving preventive screens). For women, a mammogram was the most used preventive screen (23.3% of women receiving preventive screens).

The final health behavior used in this research is social networks. The data set does not contain any overt measures of social support or social networks. As a substitute, marital status and number of children ever had was used. The average number of children reported by the respondents was 2.7 with a minimum of 0 and a maximum of 21. Marital status categories include married or cohabiting and unmarried (divorced, widowed, and never married). A slight majority of the respondents were married or cohabiting (51.8%).

Control Variables

Demographic Information. Control variables include sex, race/ethnicity, age, insurance benefit coverage, medical conditions, doctor visits and prescription medications. All controls will be measured at wave 1 to form a baseline of variables. Sixty-one point seven percent of the sample respondents were women, which is representative of this age cohort. Age was measured as exact age. The oldest respondent at the time of the first interview was 103 years old and the youngest was 69, and the mean age was 77.25 years.

Ethnic groups will consist of non-Latino Whites, non-Latino African –Americans, and Other (includes Latino, Asian and American Indian). There are too few members of other ethnic origins to form meaningful homogeneous groups with risking zero cells and unstable estimates of coefficients and standard errors. The study sample is 80.3% non-Latino White, 13.0% African-American, and 6.7% other.

Medical Utilization. A summary measure of the number of medical conditions offers a measure of the prevalence of pathological conditions, the first phase in the disablement process. The disability model focuses on the following conditions: cancer, diabetes, emphysema, heart condition, stroke and arthritis. Respondents had an average of .99 conditions. Categories of insurance coverage are: 1) Medicaid; 2) government insurance (Medicare and CHAMPUS); and 3) private pay individual plan (basic, Medi-gap, supplemental, etc.). Most of the respondents have some type of insurance coverage. Only 10% have Medicaid, but 94.2% have government insurance and a private pay plan.

As far as accessing the medical system, respondents were asked if they had had a doctor's visit in the past 12 months. Eighty-nine point two percent of the respondents had had at least one visit. The respondents were also asked the number of prescription medications they were taking. The number ranged from 0 to 20, with an average of 2.78 prescriptions. Other measures of accessing the medical system, such as hospital stays or nursing home stays or outpatient surgery were not used in this research. It was believed that these would be confounding variables, measuring the same functional limitations as the dependent variable.

Genetic Endowments. The AHEAD data set does not include any detailed information regarding genetic background, yet such information is meaningful because our genetic inheritance provides a starting point for our health in older ages and it represents our childhood environment. Long life of family members is serving as an indication of positive health genetic endowments. This research follows Smith and Kington's (1997) strategy to use substitute variables. The variables here are: 1) mother's age (if alive, or age at death), 2) father's age (if alive, or age at death) and 3) number of living siblings.

Table 3. Descriptive Statistics of Sample

	MEAN (S.D.)	PERCENTAGE	
FUNCTIONAL PERFORMANCE		Wave 1	Wave 2
Walking difficulty		37.5%	45.2%
Stair Climbing difficulty		29.8%	33.1%
Pushing/Pulling difficulty		36.7%	44.3%
Lifting difficulty		33.5%	40.1%
Picking up a dime difficulty		8.3%	11.5%
SES			
Household income ($0 - $700,000	$25,191.94 ($29,983.13)		
Net worth (-$285,000 - $14,655,000)	$182,765 ($395,668.10)		
HEALTH BEHAVIORS			
Smoking:			
Never smoked		48.2%	
Former smoker		42%	
Current smoker		9.7%	
Alcohol use:			
Abstainer		54.3%	
Light Drinker		43.6%	
Drinker		2.1%	
Exercise:			
Regular exerciser			29.3%
Diet/Nutrition			
BMI ≤18.5		3.6%	
BMI >18.5 ≤24.9		43.9%	
BMI≥24.9		52.5%	
Screenings (0 – 15)	9.47 (4.7)		
Females (0 – 15)	8.6 (4.4)		
Males (0 – 15)	10.8 (4.8)		
Social networks			
Number of children ever had (0 – 21)	2.73 (2.3)		
Married/Cohabiting		51.8%	
Education (1 – 17+)	10.84 (3.7)		
COVARIATES			
Women		61.7%	
Men		38.3%	
Non-Latino Whites		80.3%	
African Americans		13.0%	
Other (Latino, Asian, or Native American)		6.7%	
Age (69 – 103)	77.25 (5.68)		
Unmarried		48.2%	
Genetic endowments			
Father's age (20 – 107)	71.6 (15.1)		
Mother's age (18 – 109)	74.2 (17.1)		
Number of surviving siblings (0 – 13)	2.07 (2.02)		
Number of medical conditions (0 – 6)	0.99 (0.97)		
Government Insurance (Medicare, CHAMPUS)		94.2%	
Medicaid		10.0%	
Private pay insurance (Medi-gap, basic, supplemental)		94.2%	
Doctor visit		89.2%	
Prescription Medications (0 – 20)	2.78 (2.1)		

Source: AHEAD, Waves 1 and 2
a range in parentheses
b change between waves
c current age or age at death

Until sociological research and biomedical research merge data, we will not have accurate measures of genetic endowments. As a proxy, this data set includes the age of parents of the respondents. Some of the respondents' parents were still alive, so their age is reported. If the respondent's parents are deceased, their age at death is reported. In addition, the number of surviving siblings may provide some indication of the positive biological influences on health in old age. The average age for fathers of the respondents was 71.6 and ranged from 20 to 107. Mother's average age was slightly higher at 74.2 with a range of 18 to 109. The mean number of surviving siblings was 2.07 with a minimum of 1 and a maximum of 13.

Procedures

The data will be analyzed in two phases, first through a transition matrix for each functional limitation and, second, using multinomial logistic regression to analyze correlates of changes in functional status. For each of the five performance measures, there are four states that can occur over the two waves. One pair of states is stability, or no change in functional status, whether the respondent is stable with limitations or stable with no functional limitations in both waves. The second pair of states is a transition between limitations and no limitations. Recovery occurs when the respondent cannot perform the activity at wave 1, but can perform it by wave 2. Functional decline occurs when the respondent was able to perform the activity without difficulty at wave 1 but in wave 2 completes only with difficulty or no longer performs it at all. A transition matrix is an origin-destination contingency table and provides descriptive statistics of the stasis and change states in functional status of the respondents. The resulting matrix will be a 2 by 2 table for each of the measures of functional ability. This analytic step permits the description of th elevels of change, decline and recovery in the sample.

In the second analytical phase, multivariate procedures provide insight into correlates of decline, recovery and stasis. Specifically, the research will estimate the effect of SES and health behaviors on functional performance using multinomial logistic regression. This type of modeling is useful for describing the relationship between the dependent and independent variables when the dependent variable is not continuous and polytomous. In this case the dependent variable is arrayed across four categories. The categories are: 1) decline; 2) recovery; 3) stable with functional limitations; and 4) stable with no functional limitations. The basic model equation is as follows:

$$\text{Ln}[\hat{\psi}\,(\text{category 4, category1})] = \alpha + \beta_1 X_1 + \beta_2 X_2 + \ldots + \beta_k X_k$$
$$\text{Ln}[\hat{\psi}\,(\text{category 4, category2})] = \alpha + \beta_1 X_1 + \beta_2 X_2 + \ldots + \beta_k X_k$$
$$\text{Ln}[\hat{\psi}\,(\text{category 4, category3})] = \alpha + \beta_1 X_1 + \beta_2 X_2 + \ldots + \beta_k X_k$$

For each of the five functional performance measures (walking, climbing, pushing, lifting, picking up a dime), the relevant transition matrix will be used to create a four category dependent variable: maintenance of non-limited state, maintenance of functionally limited state, recovery from limited state, decline into an limited state. The reference category, category 4, is the maintenance of the non-impaired state. Three sets of contrasts are enabled: 1) decline versus maintenance of non-impaired state (category 1, category 4); 2) recovery versus maintenance of non-impaired state (category 2, category 4); and, 3) maintenance of impaired state versus maintenance of non-impaired state (category 3, category 4).

This research will estimate two regression models for each functional performance indicator. A positive coefficient indicates that a higher value of the correlate is associated with either stasis in limitation, decline, or recovery compared to maintenance of a non-impaired state. A negative coefficient indicates that a lower value of the correlate is associated with either stasis in limitation, functional decline or recovery, compared to maintenance of a non-impaired state.

The first model includes measures of SES, genetic endowments, and the covariates. The second model adds the measures of health behaviors. Comparisons of these two models describe the moderating effect of health promotion activities on the relationship between SES and functional performance. Specifically, significant SES coefficients describe a direct SES effect.

CHAPTER 4
DESCRIBING CHANGE AND STABILITY IN FUNCTIONAL PERFORMANCE

This chapter describes change and stability in functional performance. The first section presents the transition tables for each of the five performance measures. The second section evaluates the relationship of each of the correlates with the four states of each functional performance measure.

Transition Tables

A transition matrix is useful for examining changes in functional ability over time. First respondents are sorted into two categories with regards to each functional measure using the wave 1 data. The two categories are no difficulty versus difficulty in performing the function. This is the origin state. Next, it is determined if the respondents continue to have difficulty or no difficulty in wave 2. This is the destination state.

A cross-tabulation is developed with the cells on the diagonal indicating stability. That is, respondents who had no difficulty in wave 1 and no difficulty in wave 2 as well as respondents who had difficulty in both waves 1 and 2.

The upper right hand cell holds information about respondents who deteriorated over the two waves. The lower left-hand cells provide data about respondents who actually improved between waves. The cell with the largest number of respondents is the upper left hand cell indicating that the respondent had no difficulty with the functional measure in wave 1 and in wave 2. Tables 4 through 8 contain the transition matrices for the five measures of functional performance.

Table 4. Transition Matrix of Walking Several Blocks

	Destination State		
Origin State	**No Difficulty (0)**	**Difficulty (1)**	Total
No Difficulty (0)	3100.8 78.4	854.14 21.6	3954.9 100.0
Difficulty (1)	402.62 17.5	1893.9 82.5	2296.6 100.0
Total	3503.37 56.04	2748.08 43.96	6251.46 100.00

Note: Analysis used weighted data. Each cell in the transition matrix shows the cell size and the frequency percent. Source: AHEAD, Wave 1 and Wave 2

Walking several blocks. Table 4 shows that 79.9% of the respondents were stable, either with or without limitations, between wave 1 and wave 2. Forty-nine point six percent had no difficulty walking several blocks in wave 1 and in wave 2. They are shown in the upper left cell, representing stability and no difficulty, which is the most common of the cell states. The other stable state, continuing functional limitations, is shown in the lower right cell. These respondents, about 30.2% of group, had difficulty in wave 1 and continued to have difficulty in wave 2.

The upper right-hand and lower left-hand cells show the respondents who experienced a transition in functional ability between waves. Interestingly enough, 17.5% of respondents actually improved between waves 1 and 2, having difficulty performing the function in wave 1 and no difficulty in wave 2. Twenty-one point six percent of the respondents declined in functional ability between waves 1 and 2.

Climbing stairs. The transition matrix for stair climbing demonstrates similar results with walking. Approximately 79% of the respondents were stable from one wave to the next, with 75% of the stable group with no limitations, and 25% stable with functional limitations. Among the groups experiencing transition in functional ability, 16.8% declined in ability and 24.4% improved between waves 1 and 2.

Table 5. Transition Matrix of Climbing Stairs

	Destination State		
Origin State	**No Difficulty (0)**	**Difficulty (1)**	Total
No Difficulty (0)	3726.8 83.2	750.57 16.8	4477.4 100.0
Difficulty (1)	560.63 24.4	1213.4 52.8	2296.6 100.0
Total	4287.46 68.58	1964 31.42	6251.46 100.00

Note: Analysis used weighted data. Each cell in the transition matrix shows the cell size and the frequency percent. Source: AHEAD, Wave 1 and Wave 2

Pushing/pulling large objects. This functional ability parallels the results of the transition matrix for walking. Almost one-half of the group had no difficulty performing this task in either wave 1 or wave 2. Eighty-six point five percent of respondents were stable between the two waves of data, with the largest proportion of respondents being in a state of stability, no difficulty with pushing/pulling large objects (47.09%). Once again, a meaningful finding here is that almost 24.9% of respondents actually improved in functional ability between wave 1 and wave 2.

Lifting ten pounds. More than one-half of the respondents (52.3%) reported no difficulty in lifting 10 pounds in wave 1 and in wave 2. In addition, 24.8% of respondents recovered by wave 2 from the difficulty they had in wave 1 in lifting 10 pounds. Consistent with walking and pushing/pulling, approximately 21.6% of the respondents had a decline in functional ability and reported difficulty in lifting weight in wave 2 when they had no difficulty in wave 1.

Table 6. Transition Matrix of Pushing/Pulling Large Objects

	Destination State		
Origin State	**No Difficulty (0)**	**Difficulty (1)**	Total
No Difficulty (0)	2943.9 74.2	1024.5 25.8	3968.4 100.0
Difficulty (1)	568.13 24.9	1714.9 75.1	2283 100.0
Total	3512.08 56.18	2739.37 43.82	6251.46 100.00

Note: Analysis used weighted data. Each cell in the transition matrix shows the cell size and the frequency percent. Source: AHEAD, Wave 1 and Wave 2

Picking up a dime. As noted previously, the responses to difficulty with this functional ability differ from the other four. Here almost 85% of respondents had no difficulty with this function in wave 1 and wave 2 and only 4% had difficulty in both waves. Similarly to the other functional transition matrices a significant number of respondents recovered from the functional limitation. Here one-half the number who declined in ability recovered between waves of the data set.

Table 7. Transition Matrix of Lifting 10 Pounds

Origin State	*Destination State* No Difficulty (0)	Difficulty (1)	Total
No Difficulty (0)	3272.1 78.4	900.56 21.6	4172.7 100.0
Difficulty (1)	515.93 24.8	1562.9 75.2	2078.8 100.0
Total	3788.04 60.59	2463.41 39.41	6251.46 100.00

Note: Analysis used weighted data. Each cell in the transition matrix shows the cell size and the frequency percent. Source: AHEAD, Wave 1 and Wave 2

Table 8. Transition Matrix of Picking Up a Dime

Origin State	*Destination State* No Difficulty (0)	Difficulty (1)	Total
No Difficulty (0)	5281.1 91.9	464.49 8.1	5745.6 100.0
Difficulty (1)	252.45 50	253.39 50	505.85 100.0
Total	5533.57 88.52	717.888 11.48	6251.46 100.00

Note: Analysis used weighted data. Each cell in the transition matrix shows the cell size and the frequency percent. Source: AHEAD, Wave 1 and Wave 2

These transition matrices respond to the first hypothesis, that a significant proportion of older adults are free of functional limitations and some of those older adults who do suffer from functional limitations recover from them within two years. As indicated in the matrices, half of the respondents have no limitations with walking, climbing, lifting, or pushing/pulling. Over 80% have no difficulty with picking up a dime, and 50% of those who have this limitation in wave 1 recovers the ability by wave 2. Respondents had the most difficulty with pushing/pulling and lifting. Both these activities require both upper and lower body strength, and since this group is largely female may reflect their lower upper body strength. Between 17% to 25% of those who do have limitations with the other functional abilities recover between waves 1 and 2.

Correlation of Measures

Tables 9 through 13 contain the correlation coefficients of the measures used in this study. The first table, Table 9, provides the correlations among the measures of functional limitations. Functional limitations were measured in wave 1 and wave 2 and the state in each wave is compared for the correlations. A "decline" state indicates that the individual had no limitations in wave 1 but had limitations in wave 2. A "recover" state indicates that the individual had limitations in wave 1 but had no limitations in wave 2. A "stable, limited" state indicates that the individual experienced functional limitations in both waves. A "stable, no limits" state indicates that the respondent had no functional limitations in either wave. Table 10 shows the correlations between changes in functional limitations and SES measures and Table 11 between changes in functional limitations and health behaviors. Table 12 summarizes the correlations between changes in functional limitations and measures of genetic endowments and Table 13 correlations with the covariates.

Table 9. Correlation Matrix: Correlation with changes in Functional Performance Between Waves 1 and 2
Pearson Correlation Coefficients/ N=6,237

		Walking				Climbing				Pushing/Pulling				Picking up a Dime			
		(1)	(2)	(3)	(4)	(1)	(2)	(3)	(4)	(1)	(2)	(3)	(4)	(1)	(2)	(3)	(4)
Climbing	decline	.22 **	-.03 *	.06 **	-.2 **												
	recovery	.05 **	-.21 **	-.09 **	.15 **												
	stable limited	-.06 **	-.04 *	.53 **	-.43 **												
	stable no limits	-.07 *	-.07 **	-.52 **	.57 **												
Pushing/Pulling	decline	0.17 **	-.02	-.004	-.11 **	.19 **	-.04 *	-.07 **	-.06 **								
	recovery	.02	-.13 **	-.03 *	.08 **	.04 **	.-11 **	-.01	-.05 **								
	stable limited	-.04 **	-.006	.47 **	-.41 **	.002	.09 **	.47 **	.44 **								
	stable no limits	-.08 **	-.05 **	-.44 **	.49 **	-.12 **	-.12 **	-.38 **	.46 **								
Lifting	decline	.17 **	.003	.004	-.13 **	.2 **	-.03 *	-.03 *	-.09 **	.26 **	-.05 **	-.01	-.16 **				
	recovery	.01	-.12 **	-.05 **	.1 **	.01	-.12 **	-.03 *	.09 **	.01	-.21 **	-.02	.13 **				
	stable limited	-.03 *	-.02	.5 **	.43 **	.006	.08 **	.47 **	-.44 **	-.04 **	-.008	.56 **	-.47 **				
	stable no limits	-.09 **	-.05 **	-.5 **	.51 **	-.14 **	-.12 **	-.04 **	.5 **	-.14 **	-.07 **	-.49 **	.59 **				
Picking up	decline	.06 **	-.04 **	.13 **	-.14 **	.09 **	-.03 *	.13 **	-.15 **	.06 **	-.03 *	.13 **	-.14 **	.07 **	-.03 *	-.15 **	-.16 **
	recovery	.03 *	-.01	-.14 **	-.12 **	.01	-.06 **	-.12 **	.12 **	.04 *	-.04 *	-.13 **	.11 **	-.003	-.03 *	-.12 **	**.12 ****
	stable limited	-.02	-.02	.18 **	-.15 **	-.01	.01	.18 **	-.15 **	-.03 *	.006	.16 **	-.13 **	-.005	-.002	.18 **	**-.15 ****
	stable no limits	-.02	.03 *	-.27 **	.24 **	-.05 **	-.17	-.26 **	.25 **	-.007	.0005	-.25 **	.23 **	-.05 **	.008	-.27 **	**.26 ****

** p < .001 * p < .05
Source: AHEAD, Waves 1 and 2

Functional Limitations

As shown in Table 9, the changes in five functional limitations vary in the strength and significance of their correlation with one another. The strongest correlation is between the measure of being disabled in both waves. The correlation ranged from .18 between picking up a dime and walking, climbing, and lifting (between picking up a dime and pushing/pulling the correlation was .16) to .56 between pushing/pulling and lifting. This may indicate that respondents suffer from several functional limitations at one time and that they follow a similar trajectory.

The correlations of the same functional state for each measure of functional performance are, for the most part, strongly and significantly correlated with each other, except for picking up a dime. This functional performance may be fundamentally different from the other measures of functional ability. The other all involve the lower body, and pushing/pulling and lifting involves the upper and lower body with grosser muscle movements. Picking up a dime is the only measure that requires upper body mobility solely and depends on dexterity and fine motor skills. It requires more discrete movement and may indicate a more serious problem than the other measures of functional performance.

We gain additional insight by looking at each of the functional abilities on its own rather than as combined in an index. The functions have differences and shared features that provide useful information about the respondents. For example, the stable state with limitations is strongly correlated between walking and climbing (.53) and between lifting and pushing/pulling (.56). These two functional abilities share characteristics in that they use similar parts of the body. It appears that when a respondent has limitations with one functional measure they may also have difficulty with another. Limitations with walking are also strongly correlated with limitations in lifting (.5). This indicates that difficulty with walking is connected with difficulties in other functions. Additionally, the correlations demonstrate that while respondents have a tendency to have more than one functional limitation at a time, the other strong correlations are between the functional abilities in the stable state without limitations. The correlation there range from .59 to a low of .23 with picking up a dime.

Table 10. Correlation Matrix: Correlation with SES Variables
Pearson Correlation Coefficients N = 6237

		Total Household Income	Net Worth (assets-debt)
Walking	decline	-.044 **	-.046 **
	recovery	.018	.025 *
	stable limited	-.145 **	-.209 **
	stable no limits	.173 **	.238 **
Climbing	decline	-.055 **	-.064 **
	recovery	.071 **	.088 **
	stable limited	-.168 **	-.231 **
	stable no limits	.216 **	.284 **
Pushing/ Pulling	decline	-.036 *	-.046 **
	recovery	.021	.016
	stable limited	-.141 **	-.193 **
	stable no limits	.165 **	.217 **
Lifting	decline	-.064 **	-.061 **
	recovery	.042 **	.053 **
	stable limited	-.136 **	-.228 **
	stable no limits	.187 **	.271 **
Picking up	decline	-.048 **	-.072 **
	recovery	.054 **	.093 **
	stable limited	-.026 *	-.049 **
	stable no limits	.078 **	.130 **

** p < .001 * p < .05 Source: AHEAD, Waves 1 and 2

Socioeconomic Status

In Table 10, the correlations between SES and changes in functional limitations, show a significant, if modest, relationship between income, net worth and the measures of change in functional limitations. The correlation coefficients indicate that functional abilities are less likely to be limited with increasing income and net worth. Maintenance of non-limited state is correlated with higher SES. Similarly, stasis in a limited state is associated with lower values of the SES measures. Transitions are more weakly correlated with SES than static states. SES correlates more frequently with functional decline than recovery, based on the number of significant correlations. Functional declines are concentrated among lower values of SES. In contrast, higher values of income and net worth are associated with recovery.

Health Behaviors

The measures for health behavior used in this study are smoking status in wave 1 (former, current, or non-smoker), number of alcoholic drinks consumed in an average day at wave 1 (abstains, less than 1 – 2 is a light drinker, and 3 or more is a drinker), body mass index (BMI) at wave 1, participation in vigorous physical exercise three times a week in wave 2, and participating in preventive care (measured by number of preventive health care screenings for cholesterol, breast, cervical or prostate cancer, high blood pressure or a flu shot) in wave 2, social networks (number of children, marital status) and years of education. The correlations are shown in Table 11.

Stable States. The strongest and significant correlations are between the stable groups (no change in functional limitations between wave 1 and wave 2) and education, drinking, exercise and participating in preventive screens. The stable states seem more affected by health behaviors than are the transition states. Drinking behavior is measured in wave 1, while exercise and preventive behavior were first asked of respondents in wave 2. Abstaining and heavy drinking respondents are more likely to experience functional limitations than are light drinkers, those who exercise vigorously, are educated and those who engage in preventive behaviors. This is consistent with previous research that pointed to a U-shaped relationship between drinking behavior and disability (Gronbaek et al. 1998). In other words, light drinking is less correlated with health problems than is abstaining or heavy drinking.

Additional health behaviors that are statistically correlated with the stable states of most of the functional measures are weight and smoking. Being underweight or overweight is associated with increases in functional limitations, especially with walking, while normal weight is positively correlated with remaining stable with no functional limitations over both waves. Being a former smoker is positively correlated with remaining stable without functional limitations, but being a current non-smoker is not. Smoking is correlated with difficulties in walking while being a former or non smoker is more highly correlated with difficulties in climbing stairs.

Transition States: Decline and Recovery. Exercise is significantly correlated with all states of functional limitations. The association differs depending on functional ability. Thus, exercise and recovering from functional limitations go hand-in-hand, as does lack of exercise and decline in functional ability. Drinking alcohol is significantly correlated with these functional states as well. Just as with the stable group, respondents who abstain from alcohol are more likely to experience functional limitations, while those who drink fewer than three drinks per day are less likely to experience limitations.

Covariates

The covariates used in the study are sex, age, race/ethnicity, number of medical conditions, insurance coverage, doctor visits, number of prescriptions and genetic endowments. The positive, significant correlations shown in Table 13 for the stable status with functional limitations indicate this state is more likely for respondents who are female, Black, older, without insurance, have many medical conditions and visits to doctors, and are taking more medications. The opposite trends are noted for the stable status with no functional limitations.

Strong correlations are seen for stable states of walking between age and number of medical conditions. The same is true for climbing except that prescription use is also strongly correlated. Pushing/pulling stable states are strongly correlated with the respondent's sex, number of medical conditions and number of prescriptions. This may reflect women's lesser upper body strength, as lifting follows a similar pattern, with the addition of strong correlations with age. The strongest correlations among the stable states of picking up a dime and the covariates are number of medical conditions and number of prescriptions. The decline and recovery status groups follow the stable, with limitations group, but the coefficients are not as large.

Genetic Endowments. The measures here are proxies for biomedical markers. For this research the age of parents and the number of surviving siblings is used to indicate the positive health benefits passed on from one generation to the next. Parent's age is measured as the age at death for deceased parents or the current age of living parents.

Table 11. Correlation Matrix: Correlation with Health Behaviors

Pearson Correlation Coefficients N=6,237 unless noted otherwise

		Education	Non Smoker	Former Smoker	Smoker	Abstain	Light Drinker	Drinker	Normal Weight	Over weight	Under weight	Exercise N=6,235	Social network: marital status	Social network: children	Preventive Screens N=6,043
Walk	Decline	-.035*	-.004	-.009	.02	.02	-.03*	.02	.003	.004	-.02	-.09**	.03*	.03*	.02
	Recovery	.017	-.01	.006	.007	-.007	.01	-.007	.02	-.02	-.01	.03*	-.03*	-.00001	-.002
	Stable limited	-.169**	.02	-.03*	.02*	.17**	-.16**	-.04*	-.07**	.04**	.06**	-.3**	.31**	.05**	-.12**
	Stable no limitations	.189**	-.02	.04**	-.03*	-.18**	.17**	.02	.07**	-.05**	-.05**	.35**	-.32**	-.07**	.1**
Climb	Decline	-.054**	-.01	-.01	.04**	.04*	-.04**	.01	.003	-.003	.006	-.1**	.03*	-.002	-.03*
	Recovery	.082**	-.03*	.03*	.008	-.07**	.06**	.02	.02	-.02	-.006	.058**	-.07*	-.03*	.023
	Stable limited	-.196**	.04**	-.04**	.0004	.18**	-.17**	-.03*	-.04**	.01	.08**	-.22**	.27**	.07**	-.13**
	Stable no limitations	.244**	-.04**	.06**	-.02	-.2**	.2**	.03*	.05**	-.02	-.07**	.29**	-.28**	-.08**	.14**
Lifting	Decline	-.045**	.006	-.02	.02	.04**	-.04*	-.02	.0005	-.008	.02	-.097**	-.005	-.008	-.011
	Recovery	.019	.009	-.007	-.005	-.04*	.04*	.003	.008	-.005	-.008	.04**	-.07**	-.006	-.016
	Stable limited	-.126**	.1**	-.1**	-.004	.17**	-.15**	-.06**	.01	-.04**	.08**	-.24**	.27**	.06**	-.11**
	Stable no limitations	.157**	-.09**	.1**	-.01	-.2**	.18**	.07**	-.006	.04**	-.09**	.3**	-.27**	-.05**	.11**
Pushing Pulling	Decline	-.027*	-.009	-.004	.01	.03*	-.03*	-.002	.03*	-.03*	-.004	-.09**	.004	.007	-.006
	Recovery	.043**	.001	-.006	.007	-.05**	.05**	.01	.02	-.008	-.03*	.02	-.06**	-.02	-.009
	Stable limited	-.141**	.09**	-.09**	.008	.15**	-.14**	-.05**	.01	-.04*	.07**	-.24**	.26**	.05**	-.09**
	Stable no limitations	.166**	-.07**	.08**	-.01	-.19**	.17**	.05**	-.02	.05**	-.08**	.29**	-.27**	-.06**	.08**
Picking a dime	Decline	-.035-	.03*	-.03*	.005	.05**	-.05**	-.006	-.01	-.003	.04**	-.07**	.08**	-.01	-.004
	Recovery	.082**	-.01	.01	.006	-.05**	.05**	.01	.02	-.02	-001	.056**	-.09**	-.04**	.032*
	Stable limited	-.043**	-.005	.002	.002	.04**	-.04*	-.019	.01	-.02	.02	-.05**	.14**	.03*	-.02
	Stable no limitations	.094**	-.02*	.03*	-.001	-.09**	.08**	.02	.01	.004	.02	.11**	-.18**	-.03*	.03*

** p < .001 * p < .05

Source: AHEAD, Wave 1

Table 12. Correlation Matrix: Correlation with Genetic Endowments
Pearson Correlation Coefficients

		Mother's Age N=5,823	Father's Age N=5,657	# Siblings N=6,220
Walking	decline	-.01	.007	-.006
	recover	.005	-.004	.02
	stable limited	-.06**	-.03*	-.04*
	stable no limits	.07**	.02*	.05**
Climbing	decline	-.005	.03*	-.005
	recovery	-.005	.03*	.0006
	stable limited	-.07**	-.008	-.04**
	stable no limits	.06**	.009	.04**
Pushing/ Pulling	decline	-.002	.01	.02
	recovery	.01	.03*	.002
	stable limited	-.04*	-.02	-.05**
	stable no limits	.04*	.02	.03*
Lifting	decline	-.04**	-.01	-.02
	recovery	-.009	.01	-.002
	stable limited	-.03*	-.01	-.05**
	stable no limits	.05**	.03*	.05**
Picking up	decline	-.04*	-.001	-.02*
	recovery	.04*	-.008	-.003
	stable limited	-.0001	.013	.002
	stable no limits	.05**	-.01	.02

** p < .001   * p < .05
Source: AHEAD, Wave 1

Mother's age and number of siblings are negatively correlated with the measures of functional limitation (Table 12). The strongest relationship is between walking, climbing and pushing/pulling in the stable states. These tasks all require large muscle groups. Father's age is not as strongly related and is significant for the stable states in walking function and the decline/recovery in climbing stairs. All the significant correlations indicate that less functional limitations and recovery are related to increasing age in parents and higher numbers of surviving siblings.

Table 13. Correlation Matrix: Correlation with Covariates

Pearson Correlation Coefficients Number of Observations=6,237, Prescriptions N=5,262

		Respond-ent's Sex	Non-Latino White	Black	Other	Age	Medical Conditions	Insurance Plan(s)	Doctor Visit	Prescrip-tions
Walking	decline	-.007	-.04**	.04**	.01	.03*	.03*	-.02	-.004	-.002
	recover	-.033*	.003	.004	-.01	-.002	-.03*	.004	-.02*	-.02
	stable limited	.13**	-.06**	.07**	.01	.24**	.31**	-.05**	.08**	.3**
	stable no limit	-.13**	.09**	-.09**	-.03*	-.24**	-.32**	.06**	-.08**	-.03**
Climb	decline	-.009	-.03*	.02	.008	.07**	.03*	-.05**	-.014	.02
	recover	.-06**	.06**	-.05**	-.04*	-.03*	-.07**	.005	-.02	-.06**
	stable limited	.14**	-.11**	.07**	.09**	.23**	.27**	-.07**	.06**	.25**
	stable no limit	-.14**	.15**	-.1**	.1**	-.25**	-.28**	.09**	-.05**	-.25**
Pushing / Pulling	decline	.03*	-.03*	.03*	.002	.04*	.004	-.04**	.003	.004
	recover	-.05**	.03*	-.01	-.02	-.009	-.06**	.01	-.03*	-.04*
	stable limited	.23**	-.05**	.04**	.02*	.17**	.26**	-.03*	.08**	.24**
	stable no limit	-.25**	.08**	-.07**	-.04*	-.18**	-.27**	.06**	-.09**	-.25**
Lifting	decline	.07**	-.04**	.06**	.009	.05**	-.005	-.02	-.007	-.01
	recover	-.05**	.03*	-.008	-.04*	-.02	-.07**	-.008	-.02	-.06
	stable limited	.25**	-.06**	.06**	.01	.22**	.27**	-.05**	.08**	.26**
	stable no limit	-.28**	.1**	.1**	-.03*	-.24**	-.27**	.06**	-.08**	-.26**
Picking a dime	decline	.02	-.02	.03*	-.004	.07**	.08**	-.02*	.01	.05**
	recover	-.02	.06**	-.05**	-.03*	-.07**	-.09**	.07**	-.03*	-.06**
	stable limited	-.005	-.03*	.04*	-.004	.08**	.14**	-.02	.03*	.11**
	stable no limit	-.02	.07**	.07**	-.013	-.13**	-.18**	.07**	-.04**	-.14**

** p < .001   * p < .05

Source: AHEAD, Wave 1 and Wave 2

Table 14. Correlation Matrix: Correlation between all variables

	(1)	(2)	(3)	(4)	(5)	(6)	(7)	(8)	(9)	(10)	(11)	(12)	(13)	(14)	(15)	(16)
(1) Income	1.0															
(2) Net Worth	.5**	1.0														
(3) Education	.4**	.5**	1.0													
(4) Non Smoker	-.06**	-.06**	-.03*	1.0												
(5) Former Smoker	.09**	.09**	.05**	-.82**	1.0											
(6) Smoker	-.04**	-.05**	-.02*	-.32**	-.28**	1.0										
(7) Abstainer	-.22**	-.27**	-.26**	.20**	-.17**	-.07**	1.0									
(8) Light Drinker	.21**	.26**	.26**	-.17**	.15**	.03*	-.96**	1.0								
(9) Drinker	.05**	.03*	.02	-.11**	.04**	.11**	-.16**	-.13**	1.0							
(10) Exercise	.11**	.17**	.14**	-.02	.04**	-.04**	-.1**	.11**	-.009	1.0						
(11) Screens	.19**	.23**	.18**	-.09**	.13**	-.08**	-.12**	.12**	-.009	.11**	1.0					
(12) Normal Weight	.04**	.06**	.1**	.02	-.06**	.06**	-.02	.02	.002	.05**	-.05**	1.0				
(13) Underweight	-.05**	-.07**	-.05**	.01	-.05**	.06**	.05**	-.05**	-.01	-.05**	-.08**	-.18**	1.0			
(14) Overweight	-.06*	-.03*	-.08**	-.02	.07**	-.08**	-.0004	.001	.002	-.03*	.08**	-.9**	-.21**	1.0		
(15) Mother's Age	.07**	.09**	.09**	.004	-.0004	-.007	-.03*	.03*	.01	.04*	.04*	.02	.009	-.03*	1.0	
(16) Father's Age	-.01	.002	.008	.003	.003	-.009	.02	-.01	-.03*	.009	-.004	-.001	.01	-.003	.08**	1.0
(17) # of Siblings	-.05**	-.05**	-.17**	.02	-.03*	.02	.06**	-.05**	-.02*	.05**	.03*	-.03*	-.02	.04*	.03*	.09**
(18) # of Children	-.08**	-.15**	-.24**	-.03*	-.02	-.006	.09**	-.08**	-.005	-.01	-.03*	-.09**	-.006	.09**	-.03*	.01
(19) Respondent's Sex	-.17**	-.17**	-.02	.38**	.35**	-.06**	.17**	-.13**	-.11**	-.12**	-.23**	.05**	.09**	-.09**	-.04**	-.02*
(20) White	.22**	.35**	.39**	-.03*	.04**	-.02	-.17**	.17**	.004	.1**	.09**	.12**	-.03*	-.1**	.07**	-.01
(21) Black	-.17**	-.27**	-.24**	.04*	-.04**	.01	.14**	-.15**	.007	-.07**	-.06**	-.1**	.008	.09**	-.06**	.01
(22) Other	-.13**	-.19**	-.3**	.002	-.007	.009	.08**	-.08**	-.02	-.07**	-.05**	-.05**	.03*	.04*	-.03*	.003
(23) Age	-.15**	-.18**	-.15**	.16**	-.09**	-.12**	.12**	-.1**	-.07**	-.16**	-.21**	.11**	.07**	-.14**	-.05**	.02
(24) Married /Partner	.32**	.35**	.14**	-.14**	.15**	-.01	-.13**	.12**	.04*	.1**	.19**	-.02	-.05**	.04**	.04*	-.006
(25) # Medical Cond.	-.08**	-.13**	-.11**	-.06**	.06**	-.006	.12**	-.11**	-.02	-.14**	.09**	-.06**	.008	.05**	-.03*	-.007
(26) # Medications	-.03*	-.08**	-.03*	.004	.03*	-.06**	.11**	-.1**	-.04*	-.18**	.14**	-.06**	.004	.06**	-.06**	-.03*
(27) Gov. Insurance	.05**	.03*	.03*	-.02	.008	.03*	-.008	.005	.012	.007	.03*	.005	.003	-.006	.03*	.01
(28) Medicaid	-.26**	-.37**	-.35**	.02*	-.03*	.02	.16**	-.16**	-.02	-.10**	-.08**	-.07**	.06**	.05**	-.05**	.009
(29) Private Insurance	.13**	.18**	.19**	-.008	.03*	-.04*	-.08**	.09**	-.007	.05**	.1**	.03*	-.03*	-.02	.02	-.01
(30) Doctor Visit	.04*	.04**	.04*	-.005	.07**	-.11**	-.004	.011	-.02	-.04*	.25**	-.03*	-.02	.04*	-.05**	-.005

*p<.01 **p<.001

Table 14. Correlation Matrix (continued)

	(17)	(18)	(19)	(20)	(21)	(22)	(23)	(24)	(25)	(26)	(27)	(28)	(29)	(30)
(1) Income														
(2) Net Worth														
(3) Education														
(4) Non Smoker														
(5) Former Smoker														
(6) Smoker														
(7) Abstainer														
(8) Light Drinker														
(9) Drinker														
(10) Exercise														
(11) Screens														
(12) Normal Weight														
(13) Underweight														
(14) Overweight														
(15) Mother's Age														
(16) Father's Age														
(17) # of Siblings	1.0													
(18) # of Children	.08**	1.0												
(19) Respondent's Sex	-.03*	-.009	1.0											
(20) White	-.07**	-.19**	-.03*	1.0										
(21) Black	.01	.08**	.04**	-.8**	1.0									
(22) Other	.09**	.2**	-.01	-.54**	-.1**	1.0								
(23) Age	-.17**	-.07**	.08**	.007	.0003	-.01	1.0							
(24) Married /Partner	.01	-.006	-.38**	.14**	-.14**	-.03*	-.23**	1.0						
(25) # Medical Cond.	-.03*	.06**	-.03*	-.05**	.04*	.03*	.04*	-.05**	1.0					
(26) # Medications	-.05**	.02*	.07**	.01	-.009	-.007	.04**	-.03*	.47**	1.0				
(27) Gov. Insurance	.02	-.02	-.06**	-.01	.02	-.007	-.04*	.04**	.01	.00006	1.0			
(28) Medicaid	.01	.22**	.09**	-.32**	.19**	.25**	.07**	-.17**	.12**	.09**	-.06**	1.0		
(29) Private Insurance	-.03*	-.09**	.001	.22**	-.16**	-.14**	-.01	.09**	.003	.04*	-.05**	.2**	1.0	
(30) Doctor Visit	-.03*	.02	.02	-.004	.007	-.004	.009	.02	.2**	.27**	-.0006	.02	.09**	1.0

*p<.01 **p<.001

Overall Correlations

Table 14 shows the correlations between the variables used in this research. First we note that some multicollinearity exists between certain variables, such as between income, net worth and education. The resulting models may be less precise and have larger standard errors. To offset this difficulty, regression models will be estimated and tested in a step-wise fashion to determine the effects on the significance of the estimates and the standard errors. As a result, the regression modeling will use either income or net worth as an indicator of SES.

Education is used as a health behavior, as it indicates self-efficacy. Other correlations with income and net worth show a positive correlation with respondents who are White, male, married or co-habiting and of younger ages. Negative correlations among health behaviors are seen among respondents who abstain from drinking, are overweight or underweight and with increasing number of children. Among the covariates, income and net worth are negatively correlated with Medicaid, number of siblings, higher numbers of medical conditions, and higher numbers of prescriptions.

Other examples of multicollinearity exist between number of medical conditions and number of medications and net worth, education and Medicaid coverage. However, each measure adds to the theoretical basis of the model. These variables are included for control purposes and so the research is not hampered by more conservative tests of significance that may result from the multicollinearity

Indicators of the connection between education and positive health behaviors are seen here with the significant positive correlation between education and normal weight, light drinking, exercise, participation in preventive screens and former smoker, as well as the negative correlation between education and number of medical conditions. This is an additional indication that education can be used as an indicator of self-efficacy and motivation to engage in preventive health behaviors.

Response to Hypotheses

The data indicate that the first hypothesis, that a significant proportion of older adults are free of functional limitations and do experience recovery from limitations when they do exist, is confirmed by the transition matrices. For walking, pushing/pulling, and lifting, just under one-half of the respondents are free of functional limitations in both waves of the AHEAD data set and between 17% to 25%, depending on the measure of functional ability, experienced improvement in their functional status between waves. Respondents had more difficulty with pushing/pulling and lifting and much less difficulty with picking up a dime.

The second, third, and fourth hypotheses, that individuals with greater economic resources: 2) have stronger functional status; 3) are less likely to suffer decline; and 4) are more likely to recover, are also supported by the correlation coefficients. The coefficients indicate the individuals with more economic resources are less likely to have limitations in either wave. The largest coefficients are for climbing, lifting, and walking. The signs of the coefficients also indicate that greater income and net worth are associated with better functional ability, less likelihood of decline, and greater likelihood of recovery.

Likewise, the fifth hypothesis is partially supported by the bivariate data. This hypothesis is that income is a better predictor of recovery than is net worth for the transition states of decline and recovery and net worth is a better predictor of stasis states. According to the correlation coefficients, net worth is more strongly correlated with all functional states than is income. The coefficients for the correlations are larger for net worth than for income, indicating that net worth has more influence on functional limitations than does income.

The sixth hypothesis, that intervening health behaviors will modify the relationship between SES and health, will be addressed through multinomial logistic regression. However the correlation coefficients in Table 14 show us the health behaviors do vary by income and net worth. Education is strongly and positively correlated with both income and net worth. Exercising, being a light drinker and participating in preventive screens are also strongly, positively correlated with the measures of SES. The measure of health behavior with a strong negative correlation with SES is abstaining from alcohol. Other negative correlations are number of children, being underweight or overweight, being a current smoker or a non-smoker. Being a former smoker is positively correlated with SES.

Health behaviors also have influence on functional status, especially in the stable states. Education, light drinking (versus abstaining), exercise and participating in preventive screens are all positively correlated with remaining free of functional limitations in both waves, and negatively correlated with the stable state with functional limitations, especially for walking and climbing. Education, exercise and light drinking are also strongly correlated with lifting and pushing/pulling, but not as strongly correlated with picking up a dime. The presence of a social network is significantly correlated with all the stasis states, but the correlation coefficient is smaller than for other measures of health behavior. The same is true of the BMI and smoking variables. There are indications even at the bivariate level that health behaviors have strong influence on functional limitations.

CHAPTER 5
PREDICTING CHANGE IN FUNCTIONAL PERFORMANCE

Multinomial Logistic Regression Modeling

The correlation coefficients all indicate that recovery is more likely with greater economic resources, as stated in the second hypothesis. In order to determine the exact relationship as well as any intervening influences of health behaviors (the fourth hypothesis), it is necessary to look at multiple variable modeling. In this case, multinomial logistic regression modeling was used. The purpose of the modeling is to determine the maximum likelihood of obtaining the particular data that are actually observed (Power and Xie, 2000). This type of modeling is the comparison of membership in the four categories established. As a result, membership in each category is compared to the probability of membership in the reference category, in this case, being stable in each wave with no functional limitations.

Through testing the models and looking at the correlation matrices, it appeared that household income, net worth, and years of education were too correlated to use together in the logistic regression model. First, education is kept in the models because, while it is associated with SES, it is also a predictor that indicates motivation to engage in preventive behavior, which may have a different affect on health recovery. It is a measure of self-efficacy in this research and, thus, part of the set of variables measuring health behaviors. Net worth is a stronger predictor of functional ability than is household income in these models ($p<.001$). Therefore, the modeling was done using net worth as the indicator of SES and years of education as a health behavior variable.

There are two regression models. The first model tests regressing functional ability on net worth and the control variables. The second model adds preventive health behaviors, including education. The results of comparing the first and second models show that the second, saturated model is more predictive of functional limitations ($p<.001$). Therefore, the following description is of the complete model that includes the preventive health behavior variables.

Model Comparisons

Stable with Functional Limitations

Comparing the models of functional abilities illustrates the benefits of analyzing each functional measure separately. Although walking and climbing are similar, there are differences between them as among picking up a dime, lifting and pushing/pulling. This section presents comparisons of both stable states (see Table 15). The only variables statistically significant for all five functional abilities are age, number of medical conditions, and number of prescriptions, which are all control variables.

By comparing odds ratios (coefficients are reported in Appendix B), we can determine the risk of falling into the stable category with no limitations versus the stable category with limitations. A positive coefficient and odds ratio grater than 1 signals higher odds of be in the stable category with limitations A negative coefficient and odds ratio less than one indicates higher odds of being stable with no functional limitations.

Socioeconomic Status. The measure of SES, net worth, is significant for all functional limitations except for picking up a dime. The odds ratio indicates that the odds of a stable state with functional limitations is higher among the older adults with a lower net worth, especially for climbing stairs and lifting (.88). Walking and pushing/pulling odds are slightly better at .93/.92.

Table 15. The Odds Ratios of Being in a Stable with Limitations State.

	Walking	Climbing Stairs	Lifting	Pushing/ Pulling	Picking up a dime
SES					
Net Worth	.93**	.88**	.88**	.92**	.98
Health Behaviors (ref. categories: Smoking = non-smoker; Drinking = abstains; Weight = normal wt.)					
Education	.97*	.97*	1.00	.98	1.01
Smoker	2.79**	1.69*	1.64*	1.64*	1.19
Former Smoker	1.47**	1.26*	1.22*	1.05	.99
Light Drinker	.67*	.60**	.67**	.69**	.90
Drinker	.58	.41*	.28*	.36*	.30
Preventive Screens	.95**	.95**	.98	.99	.99
Exercise	.17**	.22**	.27**	.27**	.78
# Children	1.03	1.04*	1.05*	1.04	1.02
Married/ Cohabiting	1.05	1.11	1.16	1.25*	.78
Underweight	1.38	1.63*	2.12**	1.64*	1.20
Overweight	1.67**	1.37**	.83*	.83*	.87
COVARIATES					
Genetic Endowments					
Father's Age	.99	1.00	1.00	1.00	1.01
Mother's Age	1.00	1.00	1.00	1.00	1.00
# Siblings	1.03	1.01	1.00	.98	1.10*
Respondent's Demographics (referent category: Race = White)					
Sex (1=female)	1.72**	1.96**	6.48**	4.69**	.71
Black	.86	.95	.90	.75	1.27
Other (Latino, Asian, or Native American)	.61*	1.65*	.59*	.85	.40
Age	1.12**	1.11**	1.10**	1.06**	1.07**
Medical Conditions	2.09**	2.01**	1.91**	2.07**	1.63**
Utilization Issues (referent category: Insurance = Government Insurance (Medicare/CHAMPUS))					
Medicaid	1.22	1.21	1.85**	1.21	1.55
Private Pay	.75	.71	.67*	.63*	.65
Doctor Visit	.99	1.08	1.08	.96	.99
Prescriptions	1.41**	1.28**	1.28**	1.31**	1.16**
Intercept Coefficient					
Constant	-9.16	-9.81	-9.39	-6.33	-9.57
Model Log Likelihood	3689.853	3417.529	3365.676	3635.678	1430.555
N=4,977					

*p<.05 **p<.001

Source: AHEAD, Waves 1 and 2.

Health Behaviors. Exercise is the most frequent significant health behavior predictor. The odds ratio for exercise is approximately .2 for walking, climbing, lifting and pushing/pulling, indicating that those who do not exercise are 80% more likely to have functional limitations. Unfortunately the question regarding exercise was not asked in wave 1, so it is difficult to determine if exercisers are more likely to be non-limited or if the non-limited are more likely to exercise. However, this is an indication that engaging in vigorous physical activity is beneficial to maintaining functional ability.

All the preventive health behaviors are significant for the functional ability of climbing stairs, except for marital status. The highest odds ration of 1.69 is for smokers as compared to non-smokers. This indicates that smokers are 69% more likely to report difficulty in climbing stairs than non-smokers are. This is similar to the odds ratios for being underweight as compared to normal weight. There, individuals who are underweight are 63% more likely to report difficulty with climbing stairs than normal-weight older adults are. This may reflect a loss of muscle when losing weight as one ages. Similar results are seen with lifting and pushing/pulling, which may also reflect a loss of muscle mass. Social networks is another health behavior that is positively correlated with climbing and lifting limitations.

Overweight individuals have similar limitations with walking and smokers have nearly 200% more difficulty walking than non-smokers do. Walking does not require as much muscle, and lack of lung capacity may be more influential here reflected in the odds ratios for smokers, even former smokers, and overweight older adults. Persons who regularly complete preventive health screens are less likely to report walking and climbing limitations; otherwise, preventive screens do not distinguish between stability in limitations of upper body functions.

Drinking is also a significant predictor of stability in functional ability for all functions, except for picking up a dime. None of the health behaviors' odds ratios are statistically significant for picking up a dime. The odds ratios for drinking indicate that abstainers are 30 to 40% more likely to suffer functional limitations than light drinkers. These results mirror the correlation coefficients that indicate that abstaining has more negative consequences. This is also true of older adults who consume more than 3 drinks a day, which is a very small proportion of the respondents, for climbing, lifting and pushing/pulling.

Covariates. Measures of genetic predisposition included parent's age at death, or current age if still alive, and number of siblings. None of these measures are statistically significant except for number of siblings with picking up a dime. The odds ratios here are 1.10, indicating that persons who have more siblings have more difficulty picking up a dime. This is counter to the expectations that a strong genetic heritage as measured by many siblings would result in better health at older ages. This is also a change from the bivariate analysis in which a number of the correlation coefficients, especially those revealing the effects of mother's age at death, were significantly correlated with the measures of functional limitations.

Unlike the correlation coefficients in the bivariate analysis there are no significant differences between whites and African Americans. The race/ethnicity category of "Other," which includes Latino, Asian American, and Native Americans, is statistically significant, and indicate that these respondents are less likely to have functional limitations in walking and lifting than the white respondents, and more likely to have climbing limitations than white respondents. The other demographic variables that are significantly predictive are age and sex. Women are more likely than men to have walking, lifting and pushing/pulling limitations. For all functional limitations, each additional year of age raised the risk of having limitations in waves 1 and 2 by approximately 10%.

Forms of insurance are also statistically significant for certain measures of functional limitations. Limitations in walking, climbing or picking up a dime is unrelated to type of insurance. Respondents with Medicaid are more likely to suffer limitations as compared to the reference group, which has Medicare or CHAMPUS, for climbing (19%) and lifting (79%). Individuals with private pay supplemental coverage are less likely to have functional limitations with lifting (34%) and with pushing/pulling (37%) than individuals with Medicare or CHAMPUS only. It may be that this is not significant for all measures because so many of this group have some form of coverage. The presence or absence of coverage does not vary much.

From the odds ratios, it appears that the extra- individual factors of the disablement process model (Verbrugge and Jette, 1993), or the health care access and utilization factors, are the most predictive of functional limitations. Each additional prescription raises the odds by roughly 30% of remaining with functional limitations (16% for picking up a dime), and each additional medical conditions doubles the risk, holding all other variables constant.

Decline in Functional Status

This section describes the contrast between functional decline and stable with no limitations respondents (see Table 16).

Table 16. The Odds Ratios of Declining Functional Status

	Walking	Climbing Stairs	Lifting	Pushing/ Pulling	Picking up a dime
SES					
Net Worth	.93**	.90**	.90**	.96*	.93**
Health Behaviors (ref. categories: Smoking = non-smoker; Drinking = abstains; Weight = normal wt.)					
Education	.97	.95**	1.01	.96*	1.01
Smoker	1.68*	1.65*	1.7**	1.48*	1.00
Former Smoker	1.17	1.06	1.31*	1.19	.82
Light Drinker	.81*	.76*	.76*	.83*	.82
Drinker	1.47	.78	.38*	.86	.64
Preventive Screens	1.01	.98	1.02	1.01	1.04*
Exercise	.32**	.39**	.39**	.43**	.55**
# Children	1.05*	.97	1.02	1.02	.96
Married/ Cohabiting	1.19	1.18	1.19	1.22*	.92
Underweight	.74	1.52	1.69*	1.28	1.41
Overweight	1.19	1.14	.91	.81*	1.08
COVARIATES					
Genetic Endowments					
Father's Age	1.00	1.00	1.00	1.00	1.00
Mother's Age	1.00	1.00	1.00	1.00	1.00
# Siblings	1.00	1.00	.99	1.02	1.00
Respondent's Demographics (referent category: Race = White)					
Sex (1=female)	1.32*	1.15	3.05**	2.45**	1.02
Black	1.05	1.04	1.16	.98	.95
Other (Latino, Asian, or Native American)	.74	1.15	.62	.66	.64
Age	1.06**	1.07**	1.06**	1.04**	1.04**
Medical Conditions	1.53**	1.38**	1.28**	1.37**	1.35**
Utilization Issues (referent category: Insurance = Government Insurance (Medicare/CHAMPUS))					
Medicaid	.85	.73	1.02	.80	1.35
Private Pay	.82	.69	.68	.56*	.71
Doctor Visit	.85	1.18	1.16	1.17	.82
Prescriptions	1.18**	1.14**	1.09**	1.14**	1.02
Intercept Coefficient					
Constant	-5.89	-6.07	-5.71	-4.06	-5.01
Model Log Likelihood	3689.853	3417.529	3365.676	3635.678	1430.555
N=4,977					

*p<.05 **p<.001

Source: AHEAD, Waves 1 and 2.

Socioeconomic Status. The odds ratios for net worth are significant for all five measures of functional ability. Relative to the referent group, the risk of decline decreases with increasing net worth. These results are consistent across walking, climbing, lifting, pushing/pulling and picking up a dime. The difference is largest for climbing and lifting, indicating a 10% reduction in risk of functional decline for each decile of net worth.

Health Behaviors. The most consistent health behavior variable is exercise. Older adults who exercise are approximately 70% less likely to suffer from functional decline for walking, 60% for climbing lifting, and pushing/pulling, and 45% for picking up a dime. The only other variable that is statistically significant for picking up a dime is participation in preventive screens. Here individuals who did participate in preventive behaviors are more likely to suffer decline from one wave to the next (4%). Preventive screens are unrelated to other measures of functional ability.

Education is a significant correlate for climbing and pushing/pulling. Each year of education reduces the risk of decline by approximately 5%. Not smoking and light drinking are notable indicators of stability without limitations for walking, climbing, lifting, and pushing/pulling. For smoking respondents, this habit results in a greater than 50% higher risk of functional decline between waves than non-smokers experience, holding all other variables constant. Former smokers experience increase difficulty in lifting, perhaps indicating a lingering effect of smoking on functional ability. Light drinkers, on the other hand, are less likely to suffer decline by approximately 20% than abstaining older adults.

Social networks are consequential for preventing decline older adults' walking. Each additional child reduces the risk of decline by 5%. Marital status is significant for pushing/pulling indicating that married or co-habiting respondents are at greater risk for decline. Being underweight also increases the risk of decline for limitations in lifting ability as compared to normal weight respondents. Overweight older adults experience an increased risk of decline in pushing/pulling by almost 20% over normal weight older adults.

Covariates. None of the indications of genetic endowments are statistically significant here, as opposed to the results of the correlation coefficients. Demographic variables do provide some insight into additional risk factors relating to decline in functional ability.

Walking, climbing and lifting share several significant variables, respondent's sex, age, and number of medical conditions. The odds ratios indicate that women are much more likely to experience a decline between waves. For walking, they have a 32% higher risk, for lifting a 205% higher risk, and for pushing/pulling a 145% higher risk than men do. This may reflect women's lack of upper body strength relative to men's. The difference may become greater with age unless the women exercise to overcome this limitation. Correlation coefficients indicate that women are less likely to exercise (Table 14).

The odds rations for age indicate that increasing age also indicates increasing risk of decline in functional abilities. The same is true of increasing number of medical conditions and prescriptions. Respondents with more medical conditions and prescriptions are more likely to experience a decline in functional ability over the course of the two waves of the survey than respondents who are stable without any functional limitations. Race/ethnicity, insurance, and doctor visits have no significant effects.

Recovery of Functional Status

This section describes the contrast between functional recovery and the respondents who were stable, with not functional limitations (see Table 17).

Socioeconomic Status. The respondents who experienced improvement, or recovery, from functional limitations between waves are a small group and some of the patterns here are different from the previous two models. Specifically, net worth is statistically significant for walking and lifting only. For these two measures, relative to the referent group, which enjoys a stable state with no functional limitations, the risk of recovery decreases with increasing net worth.

Health Behaviors. Among the health behaviors, education is significant for climbing stairs, smoking is significant for lifting, indicating that non-smokers are more likely to recover (66%) than are smokers. Former Smoker is significant for lifting and pushing/pulling, indicating that non-smokers are more likely to recover (40%/32%) than are former smokers, once again indicating a lingering effect of smoking behaviors. Light drinkers (for climbing and pushing/pulling) are more likely to be in the stable group, as are heavy drinkers (pushing/pulling). Exercise is significant for all functional abilities, except for the measure of manual dexterity, picking up a dime. Older adults who exercise are more likely to be in the referent group, that is, they have maintained good health over the course of both waves of data.

The variable for overweight is significant for walking and climbing, which are the two lower body measures and underweight for pushing/pulling. This may reflect the differing physical demands of these activities. Walking and climbing require more lung capacity and ease of movement, and being overweight may put a strain on knee joints as well as lungs. Pushing and pulling require muscle strength, and as respondents age and lose weight they may lose muscle mass unless they exercise vigorously to maintain their muscle development.

Table 17. The Odds Ratios of Recovery of Functional Status

	Walking	Climbing Stairs	Lifting	Pushing/ Pulling	Picking up a dime
SES					
Net Worth	.94*	.96	.92**	.98	.95
Health Behaviors (ref. categories: Smoking=non-smoker; Drinking=abstains; Weight=normal wt.)					
Education	.97	.96*	1.02	.99	1.00
Smoker	1.87	1.38	1.65*	1.30	1.37
Former Smoker	1.36	1.11	1.40*	1.33*	1.23
Light Drinker	.88	.67**	.87	.61**	.75
Drinker	1.39	.61	.57	.33*	.35
Preventive	1.00	.98	.99	1.01	.99
Exercise	.50**	.53**	.6*	.63**	.83
# Children	1.03	1.04	1.02	1.04	1.04
Married/ Cohabiting	.94	1.11	.88	.93	.97
Underweight	1.62	1.09	1.34	2.30*	.77
Overweight	1.69**	1.31*	.96	1.03	1.14
COVARIATES					
Genetic Endowments					
Father's Age	1.00	.99	.99*	.99	1.01
Mother's Age	1.00	1.00	1.00	1.00	.99
# Siblings	.97	1.01	1.03	1.02	1.05
Respondent's Demographics (referent category: Race = White)					
Sex (1=female)	1.89**	1.69**	2.45**	2.79**	.86
Black	.69	1.32	1.08	.69	1.15
Other (Latino, Asian, or Native American)	.62	1.11	1.31	1.05	1.14
Age	1.04*	1.05**	1.06**	1.02*	1.08**
Medical Conditions	1.56**	1.59**	1.69**	1.80**	1.2*
Utilization Issues (referent category: Insurance = Government Insurance (Medicare/CHAMPUS))					
Medicaid	1.08	1.92**	1.41	1.3	1.81*
Private Pay	.85	1.02	1.14	.71	.42**
Doctor Visit	1.34	.86	.88	1.14	1.25
Prescriptions	1.27**	1.2**	1.18**	1.16**	1.14**
Intercept Coefficient					
Constant	-6.29	-6.08	-7.37	-3.73	-8.32
Model Log Likelihood	3689.853	3417.529	3365.676	3635.678	1430.555
N=4,977					

*p<.05 **p<.001

Source: AHEAD, Waves 1 and 2.

Covariates. The only genetic marker that is statistically significant for this group is father's age for lifting. Among the demographic and utilization variables, sex, age, number of medical conditions and number of prescriptions are important for all five functional measures (sex is not significant for picking up a dime). The coefficients and odds ratios for these variables indicate that older respondents with more prescriptions and medical conditions are more likely to be in the recovery group. Women are more likely to have functional difficulties than men are. This is indicated by the odds ratios and sign of the coefficients that point to functional limitations in wave 1 and since these variables were all determined in wave 1, it is to be expected that the sicker group would have limitations relative to the referent group.

Medicaid coverage was significant for climbing and picking up a dime. Individuals with Medicaid were 90% more likely to have functional limitations with climbing and 80% with picking up a dime in wave 1 than individuals with Medicare or CHAMPUS. Respondents with private pay Medigap insurance were less likely to have functional limitations with picking up a dime in wave 1; they were 58% more likely to be in the stable group.

The Question of Causation

One additional benefit of using longitudinal data is the opportunity to test any causal relationship between SES and health in the current period. While this research does not include any specific techniques for determining causality, it does provide information to answer the question, if we know SES in wave 1, does that help determine health status in wave 2? One test that this research can provide is to compare the model log likelihood with and without net worth included. Panel D of Table 18 shows the model log likelihood for the saturated model with and without net worth. The results indicate that net worth adds significant information to the model. We can conclude that knowing net worth helps us predict functional limitations. It adds to the argument that wealth determines health, that net worth comes first, when using functional limitations as a measure of health.

Table 18. Model Comparisons

	Walk	Climb Stairs	Push/Pull	Lift	Pick up
A. Net Worth versus Income					
	Walk	Climb Stairs	Push/Pull	Lift	Pick up
Net Worth + Education + covariates	2795.8	2760.1	2762.1	3050.3	1065.6
Income + Education + covariates	2755.2	2695.1	2728.2	2975.3	1051.7
Difference	40.6**	65.0**	33.9**	75.0**	13.9**
B. SES with Education versus Covariates					
	Walk	Climb Stairs	Push/Pull	Lift	Pick up
Net Worth + Education	437.6	602.2	344.4	490.3	116.1
Net Worth + Education + covariates	2795.8	2760.1	2762.1	3050.3	1065.6
Difference	2358**	2158**	2418**	2560**	949**
C. Health Behaviors					
	Walk	Climb Stairs	Push/Pull	Lift	Pick up
Net Worth + Covariates	2765.8	2723.8	2736.4	3038.8	1063.3
Net Worth + Covariates + Health Beh.	3689.9	3417.5	3365.7	3635.7	1430.5
Difference	924.1**	693.7**	629.3**	596.9**	367.3**
D. Net Worth					
	Walk	Climb Stairs	Push/Pull	Lift	Pick up
Covariates + Health Behaviors	3650.8	3332.9	3328.9	3574.4	1419.1
Net Worth +Covariates + Health Beh.	3689.9	3417.5	3365.7	3635.7	1430.5
Difference	39.1**	84.7**	36.8**	61.3**	11.4**

**p<.001

Response to Hypotheses

Multinominal logistic regression provides information regarding the fifth and sixth hypotheses. These hypotheses are re-stated below:

5) Income and net worth will affect functional limitations differently depending on the functional status of the individual:

    a) Net worth is a better predictor of a stable state regarding functional limitations across both waves of data. Individuals with a higher net worth will be more likely to experience a stable state with no functional limitations, while the opposite is likely to be true for individuals with lower net worth. This is due to the accumulative advantage of a higher net worth or disadvantage of a lower net worth.

b) Income is a better predictor of a transition state regarding functional limitations across both waves of data. Individuals with a higher income will be more likely to recover from functional limitations experienced in wave 1 by wave 2. Individuals with a lower income will be more likely to suffer a decline between Waves. This is due to the current onset of the disabled state and the need for more accessible resources to improve the functional status.

6) Intervening health behaviors will modify the relationship between SES and health.

Through chi-square model testing, net worth with education was the better predictor variable over household income with or without education (Panel A, Table 18) for all functional statuses. Thus, hypothesis 5a is supported and 5b is not supported. At older ages the assets that compose part of the net worth may be more liquid and available for needs. The accumulated advantage of net worth may offset any disadvantage to liquidity of the assets. Generally income declines with age and may be a less important indicator of SES.

The sixth hypothesis is borne out. The coefficients are smaller for net worth after adding the health behavior variables; Table 19 indicates the magnitude of the change in the net worth coefficients after the addition of the health behavior variables. The saturated model is statistically significantly better than the model without the health behavior variables (Panel C, Table 18). Health behaviors are tied to SES in that individuals with greater financial resources tend to be more educated and engage in more of the health behaviors. This research shows that individuals without the financial resources can affect their health through specific preventive behaviors and, perhaps, overcome the financial disadvantages they have accumulated over their lifetime.

Table 19. Net Worth Comparisons: Indirect Effects of SES through Health Behaviors

	Walking	Climbing	Lifting	Push/Pull	Pick up Dime
Decline	Yes	Small-yes	Small-yes	Small	Small
Recovery	Small	Yes	Small-yes	Small	Small
Limitation	Yes	Yes	Small-yes	Small	Small

CHAPTER 6
FOCUS ON HEALTH RECOVERY

This chapter will provide an overview of this research, address the hypotheses, and examine the usefulness of the disablement process model (Verbrugge and Jette, 1994).

Summary

This research began by questioning the health-SES connection for older adults. Does accumulated net worth and income affect the state of health of these older adults? What can we learn about these elders? Who is doing well and why? Specifically, this research proposed the following hypotheses using data from the first two waves of the AHEAD surveys.

1) A significant proportion of older adults are free of functional limitations and some of those older adults who do suffer from functional limitation recover from them within two years.
2) Individuals with greater economic resources have stronger functional status.
3) Individuals with greater economic resources are less likely to suffer a decline in their functional status.
4) Individuals with greater economic resources are more likely to recover from functional limitations when they occur.
5) Income and net worth will affect functional limitations differently depending on the functional status of the individual:

a) Net worth is a better predictor of a stable state regarding functional limitations across both waves of data. Individuals with a higher net worth will be more likely to experience a stable state with no functional limitations, while the opposite is likely to be true for individuals with lower net worth. This is due to the accumulative advantage of a higher net worth or disadvantage of a lower net worth.

b) Income is a better predictor of a transition state regarding functional limitations across both waves of data. Individuals with a higher income will be more likely to recover from functional limitations experienced in wave 1 by wave 2. Individuals with a lower income will be more likely to suffer a decline between Waves. This is due to the current onset of the disabled state and the need for more accessible resources to improve the functional status.

6) Intervening health behaviors will modify the relationship between socioeconomic status and health.

Usually we define "normal function" in terms of the performance of some "ideal of a younger able-bodied person" (Arber and Evandrou 1993: 11). As such, we have a dominant ideology that old age is a time of disability and loss of normal function. The result is problematizing old age (Achenbaum, 1996). An alternative approach is to look at aging as a process with a positive pattern. For example, in response to the first hypotheses, this research shows that a majority of elders reach their post-70 years with good physical functional ability (see Table 20).

The majority of older adults have no functional limitations and approximately 17%-24% the ones who do have limitations in wave 1do not have limitations in wave 2.

Their functions have improved between waves. However, approximately the same number of older adults experience a decline in functional ability between waves. In this research, it appears that there are several factors that influence which of these adults do well. Socioeconomic status is statistically significant. Individuals who have accumulated greater resources over their life course in the form of net worth have fewer disabilities and are less likely to experience a decline in functions over time.

Table 20. Summary of Transition Matrices

	Walking (Table 4)	Climbing (Table 5)	Push/Pull (Table 6)	Lifting (Table 7)	Pick up Dime (Table 8)
STABLE STATES					
No limitations	75.4	75.4	63.2	67.7	95.4
Limitations	24.6	24.6	36.8	32.3	4.6
TRANSITION STATES					
Recovery between waves	17.5	24.4	24.9	24.9	43.3
Decline between waves	21.6	16.8	25.8	21.6	8.1

Economic Resources and Functional Limitations

Net worth was consistently connected to the measures of functional ability. Bivariate analysis demonstrated a positive correlation between respondents with greater income net worth and functional ability. In the multinominal logistic regression net worth is again a predictor of functional ability. It appears that the accumulation of net worth over time is more predictive than current income. Income and net worth may be moving in opposite directions with age. Income drops while wealth may be at its peak.

The connection to education is interesting because education remains constant among older adults (generally), it precedes income and wealth and is not subject to reverse causation (health causing wealth rather than the other way around). Thus, education is an excellent indicator of biopsychosocial functioning in later life (Kubzansky et al. 1998). Education was used in this model as an indication of preventive health behavior, or self-efficacy. Education proved to be a consistent indicator of good functional ability at the bivariate level, but not in the multivariate analysis.

Social Policy Recommendations

Looking ahead to the growing number of elders is the opportunity to carefully consider the possible means to improve the health status of future cohorts of older adults. To improve the health of elders, just handing out money may not be the answer. Social policy could be changed to affect access, lifestyle and economics.

Access Issues

Related to issues of SES is access to medical services. Most older adults have Medicare, but still experience out-of-pocket expenses when receiving health care. Complicating the health care situation is the lack of availability of health care providers in certain areas. Expanding social programs to cover health services and to improve access could have a positive affect on the functional abilities of older adults.

Medicare does not cover such expenses as the first $600 of prescription medications, the cost of eyeglasses (except for post-cataract surgery) or hearing aids. One of the consequences of these limitations on coverage is that older adults may be attempting to function without relatively simple aids resulting in needless accidents and preventable functional limitations.

Economics

Does SES matter in the functional status of elders over time? Wilkinson (1996) points out that SES may be a proxy for social cohesion. The greater the spread between the rich and the poor the less cohesive a society is. Research has demonstrated the links between health and social networks. In a society such as the U.S. it may be that the gap between the rich and the poor is exacerbating the effect of the link between SES and health status.

There could be a significant economic return on a greater investment in maintaining and improving the functional status of retirees. If it is possible to prevent them from moving into a state of permanent or serious disability, older adults and their families could avoid requiring expensive services. Public programs such as Medicare do not cover long-term illnesses, which leaves the poor at a disadvantage.

Health Behaviors

Syme (1994) points out the importance of recognizing the environment – in this case, social class distinctions – and its influence on health. It is not just the individual's responsibility to improve health, we must look overall at the social pressures, "control of destiny" (85) and related issues in order to make a real difference in the level of health of older adults.

Health behaviors also exhibit a moderating effect on the connection between SES and functional abilities. Exercise is the most significant of these variables. Table 21 summarizes those health behaviors that are statistically significant in the multinomial logistic regression by each functional ability.

Exercise is one of the most influential activities to ensure good functional health at older ages. Individuals who exercise vigorously three times a week are much less likely to suffer from functional limitations. Linked to this is the effect of being overweight or underweight. Individuals who do not exercise lose muscle as they age. Thus, they are more susceptible to functional limitations and less likely to recover. Loss of strength is reflected in that lifting, an activity that requires upper body strength, and underweight are correlated. Social policy that offers programs for all age individuals could improve the functional abilities of older adults.

Habits learned at younger ages become a part of a lifestyle. Encouraging young adults to engage in health promoting behaviors would improve their current health status and might have positive results on their functioning at older ages. Simple educational programs aimed at school age children and more advanced programs for young adults could have a meaningful impact on future cohorts of older adults.

Table 21. Health Behaviors and Functional Abilities

	Walking	Climbing	Lifting	Push/Pull	Pick up Dime
Decline	Smoking light drinking exercise social networks	Education smoking light drinking exercise	Smoking former smoker light drinking drinker exercise underweight	Education Smoking light drinking exercise overweight	Screens exercise
Recovery	Exercise overweight	Education light drinking exercise overweight	Smoking former smoker exercise	Former smoker light drinking drinker exercise underweight	None
Limitation	Education smoking former smoker light drinker screens exercise overweight	Education smoking former smoker light drinking drinker screens exercise social networks underweight overweight	Smoking former smoker light drinking drinker exercise social networks underweight overweight	Smoker light drinking drinker exercise underweight overweight	None

Family members often serve as the gate-keeper for older adults and their access to health services and social events. Although the AHEAD data set does not have good measures of social support, there is some evidence in this research that social networks have an effect on functional ability. Social policies that support family members in their care-giving and educate them on preventive care could ensure that older adults receive appropriate and timely care, avoiding expensive and delayed care.Education regarding health behaviors is useful in helping older adults avoid problems related to high-risk behaviors. Smokers are more likely to experience decline. This may be a result of lost lung capacity. Drinking seems to follow a U-shaped curve in its connection to functional ability. Abstainers and drinkers are at more risk than are light drinkers. These results indicate that the link between preventive behaviors and functional limitations is a strong one.

Education appears to work through health behaviors in affecting functional ability. There is a reduction is the coefficients for education in the multinomial logistic regression models for walking and climbing. This indicates that education is a predictor that indicates motivation to engage in preventive behavior, which may have an effect on functional limitations that is different from the effects of SES. It is a measure of self-efficacy in this research and, thus, a measure of compliance with healthy behaviors. Any social policy that encourages continuing education and supports education at younger ages will pay benefits for older adults.

Covariates

Among the control variables, those indicating utilization were predictive as well as age and gender. Race/ethnicity was predictive at the bivariate level, but not once net worth and the indicators of health behaviors were added at the multivariate level. This may be due to confounding of race/ethnicity and SES. The more predictive indicator of functional ability is net worth at the multivariate level.

Insurance was not a strong indicator of functional ability since so many of this group have coverage through Medicare, CHAMPUS, or private plans. Prescription medications are not covered by Medicare and may be an indication of health access as well as health utilization. The more prescriptions the respondents had the higher the risk that they would also have functional limitations. Consistently, the number of medical conditions are also predictors of increased risk of functional limitations.

Why Separate Functional Measures?

In the original design of this research, a decision was made to measure each functional ability separately. The purpose was to look at each measure as a precursor to a different type of disability. While functional limitations apply to tasks or actions, according to the disablement model (Verbrugge and Jette, 1994), the next step is disability, which impinges on social roles and activities. Walking affects different social activities than does climbing, lifting, pushing/pulling and picking up a dime. In order to gather insight into the process of disablement or recovery, looking at these prior tasks could be useful as separate measures rather than as an index of function, which could blend specific problems with different functions.

Keller, Kovar, Jobe, and Brance (1993) point out the importance of consistent questioning of older adults about their functional status as well as making sure they understand the concepts of the questions. Words like "difficulty" can mean different things to different people. For someone this may mean they get a little out of breath, while another person may interpret this to mean they are in pain when they do the particular activity. Responses to "difficulty" in each of these functions may be interpreted differently by the respondents. They may have pain with walking, but climbing may result in getting a little out of breath and so they do not climb stairs or walk.

As such, these functional limitations do not always occur together and one may lead to the other. The correlation coefficients demonstrate that decline in one function is likely to be accompanied by decline in others. Examining each function on its own helps us piece together variables that affect each of these functional measures differently. However, in this research these functions have more in common than differences, except for picking up a dime. Picking up a dime requires fine pinching motion and may be indicative of a more serious medical problem. Less than 20% of the respondents had difficulty with this function.

Limitations of the Study

In measuring "health," functional limitations may be fundamentally different from traditional measures in research of the health-SES connection. Changes within two years may relate to the aging process instead (Kaplan, Haan and Cohen, 1992). A continuous variable rather than a dichotomous one may be more sensitive to detecting changes over time (Guralnik and Lacroix, 1992). The path through disease, impairment, and functional limitations may be more dynamic than is captured in the waves of data from the AHEAD survey.

One of the complications measuring functional limitations is the possibility that it is impossible to tease out the relative contribution of functional limitation due to disease and functional limitations that are a part of the aging process. The aging process includes a loss of muscle tone and a diminishment of energy (Angel, Angel, and Himes, 1992). The assumption that a cohort with a 31 year age span is comparable at all ages is similar to comparing the physical abilities of a 15 year old with a 46 year old and expecting consistency in results relating to disease and functional ability.

An additional complication is whether they are perceived to be expected limitations or whether they are due to health. Wave 2 does have specific wording to gain insight into the health-SES-functional ability connection. It may be that functional limitations are not much like disease. The social connections are more difficult to ascertain. SES may not be the explaining variable, but some other aspect of aging. How do we separate the physical limitations that are the result of the aging process from the onset of functional limitations due to the determinants of disease? The good news is that most older adults are free of functional limitations. The difference between these groups is, statistically speaking, their SES or social class.

The Disablement Model

Disablement and recovery are dynamic processes. The disablement model by Verbrugge and Jette (1994) is one attempt to standardize research into this area. It is an attempt to standardize terminology regarding functional limitations and disability and to present a clear model for research.. Verbrugge and Jette (1994) do mention steps along the process at which point prevention and intervention is useful, but they do not discuss recovery as part of their process. It seems they continue the trend to view old age as a time of continuing disability.

This research was aimed at identifying factors that help determine lack of functional limitations and even recovery among older adults. The focus was on some of the extra-individual factors that affect the second step along the process, presence or absence of functional limitations. The research also looked at stability in functional ability as well as decline. All states except stable, with no limitations, start from a point of disability. However, the trajectory to decline or recovery may be affected by SES in different ways. This research treated them the same way. The results determined that there is a range of difficulty that we can view as a range of need among older adults regarding their functional abilities.

The presence of co-morbidities are considered the precursor to functional limitations, and this group, on average, did not suffer from many medical conditions (mean = 1.0). However, the presence of other medical conditions adds to the complexity of trying to formulate a picture of the role of functional limitations and health, especially if we try to determine the relative impact of healthful behaviors. If an individual is suffering from more than one condition, complications of one condition can exacerbate the symptoms of another or treatment of the condition can result in functional difficulties. It is difficult to determine the causal relationship of risk factors to resulting limitations and disability (Fried and Wallace, 1992). Additionally, members in this study may be healthy survivors (avoiding premature death due to SES factors), but Ross and Wu (1996) found SES differences in mortality continuing well past retirement ages. Research by

Linn and Linn (1980) also found age to be a poor indicator of health among the elderly, countering the survivorship hypothesis.

This research adds to the disablement model literature by explicitly testing the relative contributions of SES and health behaviors. It appears that health behaviors can modify the SES-health link. Net worth and health behaviors represent accumulated advantage to these older adults. Future research that includes biomedical markers would help tease out the exact relationship between healthy behaviors, SES and functional ability of older adults. This type of research, blending the biological, sociological and psychological will help us understand the process of aging and ensure that the many older adults in the coming century experience a healthful old age.

APPENDIX A
SELECTED CODEBOOK SURVEY QUESTIONS

Dependent Variables

Wave 1

V852R – V882R (derived variables): Degree of difficulty walking several blocks. If need any help walking, impute a lot of difficulty.

Degree of difficulty climbing one flight of stairs. If need any help walking, impute a lot of difficulty.

Degree of difficulty pushing, pulling large objects. If need any help walking, impute a lot of difficulty.

Degree of difficulty lifting weights over 10 pounds.

Degree of difficulty picking up a dime from table.

7)No difficulty

8)A little difficulty

9)Difficulty, NA degree

10) A lot of difficulty

11) Don't do (other than for health)

12) Don't do (health reasons)

13) Can't do

Wave 2

Q1834: Because of a health problem do you have any difficulty with walking several blocks?

Q1849: Because of a health problem do you have any difficulty with climbing several flights of stairs without resting?

Q1861: Because of a health problem do you have any difficulty with pulling or pushing large objects like a living room chair?

Q1864: Because of a health problem do you have any difficulty with lifting or carrying weights over 10 pounds, like a heavy bag of groceries?

Because of a health problem, do you have any difficulty with picking up a dime from a table?

2) Yes
3) No
4) Can't do
5) Don't do

Socioeconomic Status (described in text)

Health Behaviors

V125: What is the highest grade of school or year of college you completed?

1) [0] No formal education
2) [1-11] Grades
3) [12] High School
4) [13-15] Some College
5) [16] College Graduate
6) [17] Post College (17+ years)

V298: How would you describe yourself; as a current smoker, as a former smoker, or as someone who has never smoked?

V301: Do you ever drink any alcoholic beverages such as beer, wine, or liquor? [no = abstains; yes go to V302]

V302: In general, do you have less than one drink a day, one or two drinks a day, three or four drinks a day, or five or more drinks a day?

V145: How many children have you ever had? Please don't count adopted or step-children for this question.

V150: Please remind me, are you currently married, living with a partner, divorced, widowed, or have you never been married?

BMI & Preventive Screens are derived variables and are described in the text.

Genetic Endowments

V559: How many living sisters do you have? [actual number]

V562: How many living brothers do you have? [actual number]

V565: Is your mother living? [if yes, V566; if no V572]

V566: About how old is she? [actual age]

V572: About how old was she when she died? [actual age or probe: V573; V575]

V573: Was she older than 65? [yes or no]

V575: Older than 85? [yes or no]

V576: is your father living? [if yes, V577; if no V583]

APPENDIX B
MULTINOMIAL REGRESSION COEFFICIENTS FOR FUNCTIONS

Table 22. Predicting Health Recovery in Walking
Comparison with "Stable, No Functional Limitations" Category (weighted)

	Model 1: N=5111			Model 2: N=4977		
	Decline	Recover	Limited	Decline	Recover	Limited
SES						
Net Worth	-.1**	-.1**	-.13**	-.07**	-.07*	-.08**
HEALTH BEHAVIORS (referent categories: Smoking = non-smoker, Drinking = abstains, Weight = normal BMI)						
Years of Education				-.03	-.03	-.03*
Smoker				.52*	.63*	1.03**
Former Smoker				.16	.31*	.38**
Light Drinker				-.21*	-.13	-.39**
Drinker				.4	.33	-.55
Preventive				.01	-.004	-.05**
Exercise				-1.13**	-.69**	-1.8**
Underweight				-.31	.48	.32
Overweight				.17	.52**	.51**
Social networks						
# Children				.04	.03	.03
Married/Co-habitating				.17	-.06	.05
CONTROL VARIABLES						
Genetic Background						
Father's Age	.0003	.003	-.005*	.001	.004	-.005
Mother's Age	-.002	-.002	-.003	-.002	-.001	-.003
# Siblings	-.01	-.02	.03	-.004	-.03	.03
Respondent's Characteristics (referent categories: Insurance = Medicare/CHAMPUS, Race = White)						
Sex (1=female)	.12	.48**	.47**	.28*	.64**	.54**
Black	.18	-.2	.007	.05	-.38	-.15
Other (Latino, Asian-American, Native American)	-.06	-.24	-.23	-.29	-.47	-.49*
Age	.06**	.04*	.11**	.06**	.04*	.11**
Medical Conditions	.39**	.41**	.69**	.43**	.44**	.74**
Medicaid	-.04	.26	.37*	-.16	.08	.2
Private Pay Insurance	-.25	-.32	-.47*	-.2	-.16	-.29
Doctor Visit	-.18	.31	-.21	-.16	.25	-.01
Prescriptions	.19**	.24**	.36**	.17**	.24**	.34**
Constant	-5.3**	-5.6**	-9.4**	-5.89**	-6.29**	-9.16**
	Model Log Likelihood: 2765.75			Model Log Likelihood: 3689.853		

*p<.05 **p<.001

Source: AHEAD, Waves 1 and 2.

Table 23. Predicting Health Recovery in Climbing Stairs
Comparison with "Stable, No Functional Limitations" Category (Weighted)

	Model 1: N=5111			Model 2: N=4977		
	Decline	Recover	Limited	Decline	Recover	Limited
SES						
Net Worth	-.14**	-.09*	-.17**	-.11**	-.04	-.13**
HEALTH BEHAVIORS (referent categories: Smoking = non-smoker, Drinking = abstains, Weight = normal BMI)						
Years of Education				-.06**	-.04*	-.03*
Smoker				.51*	.32	.52*
Former Smoker				.05	.11	.23*
Light Drinker				-.28*	-.4**	.51**
Mod-Heavy Drinker				-.25	-.5	-.9*
Preventive				-.02	-.02	-.05**
Exercise				-.94**	-.64**	-1.51**
Underweight				.42	.09	.49*
Overweight				.13	.27*	.32**
Social networks						
# Children				-.03	.04	.04*
CONTROL VARIABLES						
Genetic Background						
Father's Age	.003	-.006	-.0002	.003	-.006	.001
Mother's Age	.003	.002	-.002	.004	.003	.0001
# Siblings	.01	.02	.01	.005	.008	.011
Respondent's Characteristics (referent categories: Insurance = Medicare/CHAMPUS, Race = White)						
Sex (1=female)	.12	.52**	.71**	.14	.52**	.67**
Black	.11	.43*	.14	.04	.28	-.05
Other (Latino, Asian-American, Native American)	-.25	.39	.71**	.14	.11	.5*
Age	.07**	.06**	.12**	.06**	.05**	.11**
Married/Co-habitating	.19	.13	.17	.16	.11	.1
Medical Conditions	.32**	.5**	.7**	.32**	.47**	.7**
Medicaid	-.11	.77**	.38*	-.31	.65**	.19
Private Pay Insurance	-.54*	-.13	-.6*	-.37	.02	-.34
Doctor Visit	-.05	-.24	-.09	.16	-.15	.08
Prescriptions	.15**	.2**	.28**	.13**	.18**	.24**
Constant	-7.16**	-6.72**	-10.68**	-6.07**	-6.08**	-9.81**
	Model Log Likelihood: 2732.82			Model Log Likelihood: 3417.529		

*p<.05 **p<.001

Source: AHEAD, Waves 1 and 2.

Table 24. Predicting Health Recovery in Pushing/Pulling
Comparison with "Stable, No Functional Limitations" Category (Weighted)

	Model 1: N=5111			Model 2: N=4977		
	Decline	Recover	Limited	Decline	Recover	Limited
SES						
Net Worth	-.07**	-.05*	-.11**	-.05*	-.02	-.08**
HEALTH BEHAVIORS (referent categories: Smoking = non-smoker, Drinking = abstains, Weight = normal BMI)						
Years of Education				-.04*	-.007	-.02
Smoker				.39*	.26	.5**
Former Smoker				.17	.28*	.05
Light Drinker				-.18*	-.50**	-.37**
Mod-Heavy Drinker				-.15	-1.12*	-1.03*
Preventive				.01	.01	-.01
Exercise				-.85**	-.46**	-1.33**
Underweight				.25	.83*	.5*
Overweight				-.22*	.03	-.19*
Social networks						
# Children				.02	.04	.03
Married/Co-habitating				.20*	-.08	.22*
CONTROL VARIABLES						
Genetic Background						
Father's Age	-.0001	-.007*	-.001	.00005	-.008*	-.001
Mother's Age	.001	-.0005	.002	.002	.0007	.004
# Siblings	.03	.02	-.009	.02	.02	-.02
Respondent's Characteristics (referent categories: Insurance = Medicare/CHAMPUS, Race = White)						
Sex (1=female)	.77**	1.005**	1.5**	.9**	1.03**	1.54**
Black	.1	-.27	-.21	-.02	-.38	-.29
Other (Latino, Asian-American, Native American)	-.2	.25	-.01	-.41	.05	-.16
Age	-.05**	.02*	.07**	.04**	.02*	.06**
Medical Conditions	.32**	.6**	.72**	.32**	.59**	.73**
Medicaid	-.1	.42*	.33*	-.22	.26	.19
Private Pay Insurance	-.62**	-.4	-.56*	-.57*	-.35	-.47*
Doctor Visit	.09	.09	-.12	.15	.13	-.05
Prescriptions	.16**	.18**	.30**	.13**	.15**	.27**
Constant	-4.83**	-3.99**	-7.41**	-4.06**	-3.73**	-6.33**
	Model Log Likelihood: 2736.38			Model Log Likelihood: 3365.676		

*p<.05 **p<.001

Source: AHEAD, Waves 1 and 2.

Table 25. Predicting Health Recovery in Lifting
Comparison with "Stable, No Functional Limitations" Category (weighted)

	Model 1: N=5111			Model 2: N=4977		
	Decline	Recover	Limited	Decline	Recover	Limited
SES						
Net Worth	-.11**	.11*	-.15**	-.11**	-.08**	-.12**
HEALTH BEHAVIORS (referent categories: Smoking = non-smoker, Drinking = abstains, Weight = normal BMI)						
Years of Education				.01	.02	.004
Smoker				.53**	.5*	.49*
Former Smoker				.27*	.34*	.2*
Light Drinker				-.28*	-.14	-.4**
Mod-Heavy Drinker				.97	-.57	-1.27*
Preventive				.02	-.01	-.02
Exercise				-.94**	-.52**	-1.3**
Underweight				.52*	.29	.75**
Overweight				-.1	-.04	-.18*
Social networks						
# Children				.02	.02	.05*
Married/Co-habitating				.17	-.12	.15
CONTROL VARIABLES						
Genetic Background						
Father's Age	-.004	-.006	-.003	-.005	-.007*	-.004
Mother's Age	-.003	.004	.003	-.004	.005	.004
# Siblings	-.01	.01	-.006	-.009	.03	-.003
Respondent's Characteristics (referent categories: Insurance = Medicare/CHAMPUS, Race = White)						
Sex (1=female)	.98**	.88**	1.81**	1.15**	.9**	1.87**
Black	.21	.03	-.06	.15	.08	-.11
Other (Latino, Asian-American, Native American)	-.37	.27	-.34	-.48	.27	-.52*
Age	.06**	.06**	.11**	.06**	.06**	.09**
Medical Conditions	.25**	.53**	.64**	.25**	.52**	.65**
Medicaid	.05	.37	.72**	.02	.34	.61**
Private Pay Insurance	-.36	.15	-.53*	-.39	.13	-.4*
Doctor Visit	.17	-.2	-.02	.15	-.16	.07
Prescriptions	.13**	.19**	.3**	.09**	.15**	.27**
Constant	-5.5**	-7.4**	-10.3**	-5.71**	-7.37**	-9.39**
	Model Log Likelihood: 3038.81			Model Log Likelihood: 3635.678		

*p<.05 **p<.001

Source: AHEAD, Waves 1 and 2.

Table 26. Predicting Health Recovery in Picking Up a Dime
Comparison with "Stable, No Functional Limitations" Category (weighted)

	Model 1: N=5111			Model 2: N=4977		
	Decline	Recover	Limited	Decline	Recover	Limited
SES						
Net Worth	-.08**	-.08*	-.03	-.08**	-.05	-.02
HEALTH BEHAVIORS (referent categories: Smoking = non-smoker, Drinking = abstains, Weight = normal BMI)						
Years of Education				.006	.004	-.01
Smoker				-.004	.32	.18
Former Smoker				-.19	.21	.005
Light Drinker				-.2	-.29	-.1
Mod-Heavy Drinker				-.45	-1.05	-1.19
Preventive				.04*	-.02	-.01
Exercise				-.6**	-.19	-.24
Underweight				.34	-.27	.18
Overweight				.08	.12\3	-.14
Social networks						
# Children				-.04	.04	.02
Married/Co-habitating	-.1	-.03	-.19	-.08	-.03	-.25
CONTROL VARIABLES						
Genetic Background						
Father's Age	.001	-.002	.007	.001	-.007	.007
Mother's Age	-.004	-.008*	.001	-.005	-.007	.002
# Siblings	.007	.06	.1*	.001	.05	.1*
Respondent's Characteristics (referent categories: Insurance = Medicare/CHAMPUS, Race = White)						
Sex (1=female)	.06	-.06	-.22	.02	-.15	-.34
Black	-.01	.16	.21	-.05	.14	.24
Other (Latino, Asian-American, Native American)	-.43	.13	-1.0*	-.45	.13	-.91
Age	.04**	.08**	.08**	.04**	.08**	.07**
Medical Conditions	.3**	.22*	.49**	.3**	.18*	.49**
Medicaid	.28	.55*	.49*	.3	.59*	.44
Private Pay Insurance	-.29	-.96**	-.35	-.35	-.88**	-.43
Doctor Visit	-.06	.3	-.02	-.2	.23	-.005
Prescriptions	.05	.12**	.16**	.02	.13**	.15**
Constant	-5.5**	-8.27**	-10.6**	-5.01**	-8.32**	-9.57**
	Model Log Likelihood: 1063.28			Model Log Likelihood: 1430.555		

*p<.05 **p<.001

Source: AHEAD, Waves 1 and 2.

LIST OF REFERENCES

Achenbaum, W. Andrew. 1996. "Historical Perspectives on Aging." Pp. 137 – 152 in *Handbook of Aging and the Social Sciences*. Robert H. Binstock and Linda George eds. Washington, D.C.: Academic Press.

Adler, Nancy, Thomas Boyce, Margaret Chesney, Sheldon Cohen, Susan Folkman, Robert Kahn, Leonard Syme. 1994. "Socioeconomic Status and Health: The Challenge of the Gradient." *American Psychologist*. 49(1)15-24.

Angel, Ronald and Jacqueline Angel. 1996. "The Extent of Private and Public Health Insurance Coverage Among Adult Hispanics." *The Gerontologist*. 36(3):332-340.

Angel, Ronald, Jacqueline Angel and Christine Himes. 1992. "Minority Group Status, Health Transitions, and Community Living Arrangements Among the Elderly." *Reasearch on Aging*. 14(4): 496-521.

Arber, Sara and Maria Evandrou. 1993. "Mapping the Territory." Pp. 9 – 26 in *Ageing, Independence and the Life Course*. Sara Arber and Maria Evandrou, editors. London: Jessica Kingsley Publishers.

Arber, Sara and Helen Cooper. 1999. "Gender Differences in Health in Later Life: the New Paradox?" *Social Science & Medicine*. 48:61-76.

Arber, Sara and Jay Ginn. 1993. "Gender and Inequalities in Health in Later Life." *Social Science and Medicine*. 36(1):33-46.

Arber, Sara and Jay Ginn, 1991. "The Invisibility of Age: Gender and Class in Later Life." *The Sociological Review*. 39(2):260-291.

Atchley, Robert. 1998. "Activity Adaptations to the Development of Functional Limitations and Results for Subjective Well-being in Later Adulthood: a Qualitative Analysis of Longitudinal Panel Data over a 16-Year Period." *Journal of Aging Studies*. 12(1):19 – 39.

Beckett, Laurel, Dwight Brock, Jon Lemke, Carlos Mendes de Leon, Jack Guralnik, Gerda Fillenbaum, Laurence Branch, Terrie Wetle, and Denis Evans. 1996. "Analysis of Change in Self-reported Physical Function among Older Persons in Four Population Studies." *American Journal of Epidemiology*. 143(6):766-778.

Beckett, Megan. 2000. "Converging Health Inequalities in Later Life—an Artifact of Mortality Selection?" *Journal of Health and Social Behavior*. 41(1):106-119.

Bennett, Kate and Kevin Morgan. 1993. "Ageing, Gender and the Organisation of Physical Activities." Pp. 78 – 90 in *Ageing, Independence and the Life Course*. Sara Arber and Maria Evandrou, editors. London: Jessica Kingsley Publishers.

Berkman, Lisa and Jewel Mullen. 1997. "How Health Behaviors and the Social Environment Contribute to Health Differences Between Black and White Older Americans." Pp. 163 – 182 in *Racial and Ethnic Differences in the Health of Older Americans*. Linda Martin and Beth Soldo, editors. Washington, D.C.: National Academy Press.

Berkman, Lisa, Thomas Oxman, and Teresa Seeman. 1992. "Social Networks and Social Support Among the Elderly: Assessment Issues." Pp. 196 – 212 in *The Epidemiologic Study of the Elderly*. Robert Wallace and Robert Woolson, eds. New York: Oxford University Press.

Bound, John, Michael Schoenbaum and Timothy Waidmann. 1995. "Race and Education Differences in Disability Status and Labor Force Attachment in the Health and Retirement Survey." *The Journal of Human Resources* (Supplement). 30:S227-S267.

Brown, Charles. 1996. "Symposium II: Income and Wealth." *The Gerontologist*. 36(3):341.

Cartwright, William S. 1992. "Assessing Income and Resources of the Elderly." Pp. 281 – 286 in *Epidemiologic Study of the Elderly*. Robert Wallace and Robert Woolson, eds. New York: Oxford University Press.

Charmaz, Kathy. 1995. "The Body, Identity, and Self: Adapting to Impairment." *The Sociological Quarterly*. 36:657-680.

Chirikos, Thomas and Jennie Nickel. 1986. "Socioeconomic Determinants of Continuing Functional Disablement from Chronic Disease Episodes." *Social Science & Medicine*. 22(12):1329-1335.

Choudhury, Sharmila and Michael Leonesio. 1997. "Life-Cycle Aspects of Poverty Among Older Women." *Social Security Bulletin*. 60(2):17-37.

Clark, Daniel, Christopher Callahan, Simon Mungai, Frederic Wolinsky. 1996. "Physical Function Among Retirement-Aged African American Men and Women." *The Gerontologist*. 36(3):322-331.

Council on Scientific Affairs, American Medical Association. 1996 "Alcoholism in the Elderly". *JAMA*. 275(10):797-802.

Cress, M. Elaine, David Buchner, Kent Questad, Peter Esselman, Barbara deLateur, and Robert Schwartz. 1999. "Exercise: Effects on Physical Functional Performance in Independent Older Adults." *Journal of Gerontology: Medical Sciences*. 54A(5):M242-M248.

Crimmins, Eileen. 1996. "Mixed Trends in Population Health Among Older Adults." *Journal of Gerontology: Social Sciences*. 51B:S223-S225.

Crimmins, Eileen. 1997. "Trends in Disability-Free Life Expectancy in the United States: 1970 – 1990." *Population and Development Review*. 23(3):555-573.

Crystal, Stephen. 1996. "Economic Status of the Elderly." Pp. 388 – 409 in *Handbook of Aging and the Social Sciences*. Robert H. Binstock and Linda George eds. Washington, D.C.: Academic Press.

Daltroy, Lawren, Martin Larson, Holley Eaton, Charlotte Phillips, Matthew Liang. 1999. "Discrepancies between Self-Reported and Observed Physical Function in the Elderly: the Influence of Response Shift and Other Factors." *Social Science & Medicine*. 48:1549-1561.

Deaton, Angus and Christina Paxson. 1998. "Aging and Inequality in Income and Health." *American Economic Review*. 88(2):248-254.

Elo, Irma and Samuel Preston. 1996. "Education Differentials in Mortality: United State, 1979-85. *Social Science & Medicine*. 42(1):47-57.

Estes, Carroll. 1989. "Aging, Health and Social Policy: Crisis and Crossroads." *Journal of Aging & Social Policy*. 1(1/2):17-32.

Evandrou, Maria and Jane Falkingham. 1993. "Social Security and the Life Course: Developing Sensitive Policy Alternatives." Pp. 201 – 223 in *Ageing, Independence and the Life Course*. Sara Arber and Maria Evandrou, editors. London: Jessica Kingsley Publishers.

Feinstein, Jonathan S. 1993. "The Relationship Between Socioeconomic Status And Health: A Review Of The Literature." *The Milbank Quarterly*. 71(2):279-323.

Ferraro, Kenneth. 1993. "Are Black Older Adults Health-Pessimistic?" *Journal of Health and Social Behavior*. 34:201-214.

Ferraro, Kenneth and Melissa Farmer. 1996. "Double Jeopardy, Aging as Leveler, or Persistent Health Inequality? A Longitudinal Analysis of White and Black Americans." *Journal of Gerontology: Social Sciences*. 51B(6):S319-S328.

Freedman, Vicki and Linda Martin. 1998. "Understanding Trends in Functional Limitations Among Older Americans." *American Journal of Public Health.* 88(10):1457-1462.

Fried, Linda and Robert Wallace. 1992. "The Complexity of Chronic Illness in the Elderly: from Clinic to Community." Pp. 10 – 19 in *The Epidemiologic Study of the Elderly.* New York: Oxford University Press.

Fries, James. 1989 "The Compression of Morbidity: Near or Far?" *The Milbank Quarterly.* 65(2):208-233.

Fry, Christine. 1996. "Age, Aging, and Culture." Pp. 117 – 136 in *Handbook of Aging and the Social Sciences, 4th ed.* Robert Binstock and Linda George, eds. San Diego: Academic Press.

George, Linda. 1996. "Social Factors and Illness." Pp. 229 – 252 in *Handbook of Aging and the Social Sciences, 4th ed.* Robert Binstock and Linda George, eds. San Diego: Academic Press.

Goldman, Noreen, Sanders Korenman and Rachel Weinstein. 1995. "Marital Status and Health Among the Elderly." *Social Science & Medicine.* 40(12):1717-1730.

Gronbaek, Morten, Allan Deis, Ulrik Becker, Hans Ole Hein, Peter Schnohr, Gorm Jensen, Knut Borch-Johnson, and Thorkild Sorensen. 1998. "Alcohol and Mortality: Is There a U-Shaped Relation in Elderly People?" *Age and Ageing.* 27(6)739-744.

Guccione, Andrew, David Felson, Jennifer Anderson, John Anthony, Yuqing Zhang, Peter Wilson, Margaret Kelly-Hayes, Philip Wolf, Bernard Kreger, and William Kannel. 1994. "The Effects of Specific Medical Conditions on the Functional Limitations of Elders in the Framingham Study." *American Journal of Public Health.* 84(3):351-358.

Guralnik, Jack and Andrea Lacroix. 1992. "Assessing Physical Function in Older Populations." Pp. 159 – 181 in *The Epidemiologic Study of the Elderly.* Robert Wallace and Robert Woolson, eds. New York: Oxford University Press.

Guralnik, Jack M., Kenneth Land, Dan Blazer, Gerda Fillenbaum, and Laurence Branch. 1993. "Educational Status and Active Life Expectancy Among Older Blacks and Whites." *The New England Journal of Medicine.* 329(2):110-117.

Harwood, Rowan, Martin Prince, Anthony Mann and Shah Ebrahim. 1998. "Associations Between Diagnoses, Impairments, Disability and Handicap in a Population of Elderly People." *International Journal of Epidemiology.* 27:261-268.

House, James, James Lepkowski, Ann Kinney, Richard Mero, Ronald Kessler, and Regula Herzog. 1994. "The Social Stratification of Aging and Health." *Journal of Health and Social Behavior.* 35:213-234.

Howarth, Glennys. 1993. "Good Consumption, Social Roles and Personal Identity." Pp. 65 – 77 in *Ageing, Independence and the Life Course.* Sara Arber and Maria Evandrou, editors. London: Jessica Kingsley Publishers.

Jette, Alan M. 1996. "Disability Trends and Transitions." Pp. 94 – 116 in *Handbook of Aging and the Social Sciences, 4th ed.* Robert Binstock and Linda George, eds. San Diego: Academic Press.

Jette, Alan. 1999. "Disentangling the Process of Disablement." *Social Science and Medicine.* 48:471-472.

Jette, Alan M., Sybil Crawford and Sharon Tennstedt. 1996. "Toward Understanding Ethnic Differences in Late-Life Disability." *Research on Aging.* 18(3): 292-309.

Johnson, Robert and Frederic Wolinsky. 1993. "The Structure of Health Status among Older Adults: Disease, Disability, Functional Limitation, and Perceived Health." *Journal of Health and Social Behavior.* 34(2):105-121.

Johnson, Robert and Fredric Wolinsky. 1994. "Gender, Race, and Health: The Structure of Health Status Among Older Adults." *The Gerontologist.* 34(1):24-35.

Kaplan, George, Mary Haan, and Richard Cohen. 1992 "Risk Factors and the Study of Prevention in the Elderly: Methodological Issues." Pp. 20 – 38 in *The Epidemiologic Study of the Elderly.* Robert Wallace and Robert Woolson, eds. New York: Oxford Press.

Katz, Mitchell. 1999. *Multivariable Analysis: A Practical Guide for Clinicians.* New York: Cambridge University Press.

Keller, Donald, Mary Grace Kovar, Jared Jobe, Laurence Branch. 1993. "Problems Eliciting Elders' Reports of Functional Status." *Journal of Aging and Health.* 5(3):306-318.

Kington, Raynard and James Smith. 1997. "Socioeconomic Status and Racial and Ethnic Differences in Functional Status Associated with Chronic Diseases." *American Journal of Public Health.* 87(5):805-810.

Kubzansky, Laura, Lisa Berkman, Thomas Glass, and Teresa Seeman. 1998. "Is Educational Attainment Associated with Shared Determinants of Health in the Elderly? Findings from the MacArthur Studies of Successful Aging." *Psychosomatic Medicine.* 60:578-585.

Linn, Bernard and Margaret Linn. 1980. "Objective and Self-Assessed Health in the Old and Very Old." *Social Science & Medicine.* 14A:311-315.

Link, Bruce and Jo Phelan. 1995. "Social Conditions as Fundamental Causes of Disease." *Journal of Health and Social Behavior* (Extra Issue):80-94.

Lynch, John, George Kaplan, and Sarah Shema. 1997. "Cumulative Impact of Sustained Economic Hardship on Physical, Cognitive, Psychological, and Social Functioning." *New England Journal of Medicine.* 337(26):1889-1895.

Manton, Kenneth and Eric Stallard. 1996. "Changes in Health, Mortality, and Disability and Their Impact on Long-Term Care Needs." *Journal of Aging & Social Policy.* 7(3/4):25-52.

Markides, Kyriakos, David Lee, Laura Ray, and Sandra Black. 1993. "Physicians' Ratings of Health in Middle and Old Age: A Cautionary Note." *Journal of Gerontology: Social Sciences.* 48(1):S24-S27.

Markides, Kyriakos, Laura Rudkin, Ronald Angel, and David Espino. 1997. "Health Status of Hispanic Elderly." Pp. 285-300 in *Racial and Ethnic Differences in the Health of Older Americans.* Linda Martin and Beth Soldo, Eds. Washington D.C.: National Academy Press.

Marmot, Michael, Rebecca Fuhrer, Susan Ettner, Nadine Marks, Larry Bumpass and Carol Ryff. 1998. "Contribution of Psychosocial Factors to Socioeconomic Differences in Health." *The Milbank Quarterly.* 76(3):403-448.

McBride, Judy. 1992. "Lean on Me: Understanding Age-Related Loss of Muscle Tissue." *Agricultural Research.* 40(5):17-20.

Mechanic, David. 1995. "Sociological Dimensions of Illness Behavior." *Social Science and Medicine.* 41 (9):1207-1216.

Menard, Scott. 1995. *Applied Logistic Regression Analysis.* Sage University Paper series on Quantitative Applications in the Social Sciences, 07-106. Thousand Oaks, CA: Sage.

Mendes de Leon, Carlos, Laurel Beckett, Gerda Fillenbaum, Dwight Brock, Laurence Branch, Denis Evans, and Lisa Berkman. 1997. "Black-White Differences in Risk of Becoming Disabled and Recovering from Disability in Old Age: A Longitudinal Analysis of Two EPESE Populations." *American Journal of Epidemiology.* 145(6):488-497.

Mirowsky, John. 1998. "Education, Personal Control, Lifestyle and Health: A Human Capital Hypothesis." *Research on Aging.* 20(4):415-450.

Mirowsky, John and Paul Nongzhuang Hu. 1996. "Physical Impairment and the Diminishing Effects of Income." *Social Forces*. 74(3):1073-1096.

Mirowsky, John and Catherine Ross. 1999. "Economic Hardship Across the Life Course." *American Sociological Review*. 64(August):548-569.

Moen, Phyllis, Donna Dempster-McClain, and Robin Williams, Jr. "Successful Aging: A Life-Course Perspective on Women's Multiple Roles and Health." *American Journal of Sociology*. 97(6):1612-1638.

Moore, Alison, Sally Morton, John Beck, Ron Hays, Sabine Oishi, Jennifer Partridge, Barbara Genovese, and Arlene Fink. 1999. "A New Paradigm for Alcohol Use in Older Persons." *Medical Care*. 37(2):165-179.

Morris, Shirley, Sylvia Sherwood and John Morris. 1996. "A Dynamic Model for Explaining Changes in Use of IADL/ADL Care in the Community." *Journal of Health and Social Behavior*. 37(March):91-103.

Myers, George, F. Thomas Juster, and Richard Suzman. 1997. "Introduction." *The Journal of Gerontology* (Special Issue). 52B:v-viii.

Nagi, Saad. 1976. "An Epidemiology of Disability among Adults in the United States." *Milbank Memorial Fund Quarterly*. 54:439-468.

O'Rand, Angela. 1996. "The Cumulative Stratification of the Life Course." Pp. 188 – 207 in *Handbook of Aging and the Social Sciences, 4th edition*. Robert Binstock and Linda George, editors. San Diego: Academic Press.

O'Rand, Angela and John Henretta. 1999. *Age and Inequality: Diverse Pathways Through Later Life*. Boulder: Westview Press.

Powers, Daniel A and Yu Xie. 2000. *Statistical Methods for Categorical Data Analysis*. San Diego: Academic Press.

Preston, Samuel and Paul Taubman. 1994. "Socioeconomic Differences in Adult Mortality and Health Status." *Demography of Aging*. L.G. Martin and S.H. Preston, eds. Washington, D.C.: Academic Press.

Reynolds, John and Catherine Ross. 1998. "Social Stratification and Health: Education's Benefit Beyond Economic Status and Social Origins." *Social Problems*. 45(2):221-247.

Rogers, Richard. 1995. "Sociodemographic Characteristics of Long-Lived and Healthy Individuals." *Population and Development Review*. 21(1):33-59.

Ross, Catherine and Chia-Ling Wu. 1996. "Education, Age, and the Cumulative Advantage in Health." *Journal of Health and Social Behavior*. 37(March):104-120.

Ruchlin, Hirsch and Mark Lachs. 1999. "Prevalence and Correlates of Exercise Among Older Adults." *The Journal of Applied Gerontology*. 18(3):341-357.

Scheidt, Rick, Daniel Humpherys, and Jeremy Yorgason. 1999. "Successful Aging: What's Not to Like?". *The Journal of Applied Gerontology*. 18 (3): 277-282.

Smith, James. 1995. "Unequal Wealth and Incentives to Save." RAND. Santa Monica, California: RAND.

Smith, James. 1997. "Wealth Inequality Among Older Americans." *The Journals of Gerontology*. 52B:74-81.

Smith, James and Raynard Kington. 1997a. "Demographic and Economic Correlates of Health in Old Age." *Demography*. 34:159-170.

Smith, James and Raynard Kington. 1997b. "Race, Socioeconomic Status, and Health." Pp. 105-062 in *Racial and Ethnic Differences in the Health of Older Americans*. Linda Martin and Beth Soldo, editors. Washington, D.C.: National Academy Press.

Soldo, Beth, Michael Hurd, Willard Rodgers, and Robert Wallace. 1997. "Asset and Health Dynamics Among the Oldest Old: An Overview of the AHEAD Study." *The Journals of Gerontology* (Special Issue). 52B:1-20.

Stevens, June, Jiawen Cai, Elsie Pamuk, David Williamson, Michael Thun, Joy Wood. 1998. "The Effect of Age on the Association between Body-Mass Index and Mortality." *New England Journal of Medicine*. 338(1):1-7.

Stoller, Eleanor. 1994. "Factors Affecting the Frequency of Health Enhancing Behaviors by The Elderly." *Public Health Reports*. 109(3):377-390.

Straus, Robert. 1999. "Medical Sociology: A Personal Fifty Year Perspective." *Journal of Health and Social Behavior*. 40(June):103-110.

Syme, Leonard. 1994. "The Social Environment and Health." *Daedalus*. 123(4):79-86.

Thorslund, Mat and Lundberg Ole. 1994. "Health Inequalities Among the Oldest Old." *Journal of Aging and Health*. 6:51-69.

Turner, Bryan S. 1984. *The Body and Society*. Oxford, UK: Basil Blackwell Publisher, Ltd.

Uhlenberg, Peter and Sonia Miner. 1996. "Life Course and Aging: A Cohort Perspective." Pp. 208 – 228 in *Handbook of Aging and the Social Sciences, 4th edition.* Robert Binstock and Linda George, editors. San Diego: Academic Press.

U.S. Bureau of the Census. 1996. "65+ in the United States." *Current Population Reports, Special Studies*, 23-190. Washington, D.C.: U.S. Government Printing Office.

Verbrugge, Lois and Alan M. Jette. 1994. "The Disablement Process." *Social Science and Medicine.* 38(1):1-14.

Verbrugge, Lois, Joseto Reoma, and Ann Gruber-Baldini. 1994. "Short-Term Dynamics of Disability and Well-Being. " *Journal of Health and Social Behavior.* 35(June):97-117.

Visser, M., T.B. Harris, J. Langlois, M.T. Hannan, R. Roubenoff, D.T. Felson, P.W.F. Wilson, D.P. Kiel. 1998. "Body Fat and Skeletal Muscle Mass in Relation to Physical Disability in Very Old Men and Women of the Framingham Heart Study." *The Journals of Gerontology, Series A.* 53(3):M214-M222.

Waldron, Ingrid and Jerry Jacobs. 1988. "Effects of Labor Force Participation on Women's Health: New Evidence from a Longitudinal Study." *Journal of Occupational Medicine.* 30:977-983.

Wallace, Robert. 1992. "Aging and Disease: From Laboratory to Community." Pp. 3 – 9 in *The Epidemiologic Study of the Elderly.* Robert Wallace and Robert Woolson, editors. New York: Oxford Press.

Wiener, Joshua and Laurel Illston. 1996 "The Financing and Organization of Health Care for Older Americans. Pp. 427 – 445 in *Handbook of Aging and the Social Sciences, 4th edition.* Robert Binstock and Linda George, editors. San Diego: Academic Press.

Whitfield, Keith and Tamara Baker-Thomas. 1999. "Individual Differences in Aging Minorities." *International Journal of Aging and Human Development.* 48(1):73-79.

Wilkinson, Doris. 1988. "Mother-Daughter Bonds in the Later Years: Transformation of the 'Help Pattern.'" in *Family and Support Systems Across the Life Span.* Suzanne K. Steinmetz, editor.

Wilkinson, Richard. 1996. *Unhealthy Societies: The Affliction of Inequality.* New York: Routledge.

Wilcox-Gők, Virginia and Jeffrey Rubin. 1994. "Health Insurance Coverage Among the Elderly." *Social Science & Medicine.* 38(11):1521-1529.

Wilson, Gail. 1993. "Money and Independence in Old Age." Pp. 46 - 64 in *Ageing, Independence and the Life Course*. Sara Arber and Maria Evandrou, editors. London: Jessica Kingsley Publishers.

Wolinsky, Fredric, Timothy Stump, Christopher Callahan, and Robert Johnson. 1996. "Consistency and Change in Functional Status Among Older Adults Over Time." *Journal of Aging and Health*. 8(2):155-182.

BIOGRAPHICAL SKETCH

An Army "brat," Dorothy McCawley was born in Anchorage, Alaska, and subsequently lived in five states and two other countries. Being exposed to a variety of cultures piqued Ms. McCawley's interest in understanding the dynamics of group behavior. Once her father retired from the military service, the family settled in Gainesville, Florida, where they had family connections.

After high school, Ms. McCawley pursued a career in the health care profession as an ophthalmic technologist. There she gained an insider's view of the United States health care system and a provider's perspective. However, vertical advancement is limited as a technologist, so, in an effort to expand her career horizon, Ms. McCawley returned to the University of Florida earning joint advanced degrees, the Master in Business Administration and Master in Health Service Administration. After nearly a year with the Veterans Administration, Ms. McCawley pursued a career as an entrepreneurial capitalist. As owner of Fringe Benefit Coordinators, Inc., she learned about the insurance side of the health care system.

In the meantime, Ms. McCawley continued to aspire to enlightenment and received a master's in pastoral studies from Loyola University, New Orleans, through a distance learning program. In a desire to unify her life experiences and her educational attainment, Ms. McCawley then decided to work towards a doctoral degree in sociology. Sociology seemed to be the ideal discipline to provide a means to advance her understanding of the world she had experienced growing up and working in as well as additional insight into the non-obvious aspects of social experiences.

At this time, Ms. McCawley continues as owner and President of Fringe Benefit Coordinators, Inc., and is an adjunct faculty member at the Santa Fe Community College and teaches courses for the Diocese of St. Augustine. She looks forward to a long life of learning and expanding her horizons and doting on her five nieces and nephews. Her philosophy of life is "Use it or lose it!" and in that vein she will continue to use her mind and will share with others the riches of sociological insight.

I certify that I have read this study and that in my opinion it conforms to acceptable standards of scholarly presentation and is fully adequate, in scope and quality, as a dissertation for the degree of Doctor of Philosophy.

Barbara A. Zsembik, Chair
Associate Professor of Sociology

I certify that I have read this study and that in my opinion it conforms to acceptable standards of scholarly presentation and is fully adequate, in scope and quality, as a dissertation for the degree of Doctor of Philosophy.

Donna H. Berardo, Cochair
Associate Professor of Sociology
Pharmacy Health Care Administration

I certify that I have read this study and that in my opinion it conforms to acceptable standards of scholarly presentation and is fully adequate, in scope and quality, as a dissertation for the degree of Doctor of Philosophy.

Leonard Beeghley
Professor of Sociology

I certify that I have read this study and that in my opinion it conforms to acceptable standards of scholarly presentation and is fully adequate, in scope and quality, as a dissertation for the degree of Doctor of Philosophy.

Charles W. Peek
Assistant Professor of Sociology

I certify that I have read this study and that in my opinion it conforms to acceptable standards of scholarly presentation and is fully adequate, in scope and quality, as a dissertation for the degree of Doctor of Philosophy.

Otto von Mering
Professor of Anthropology

This dissertation was submitted to the Graduate Faculty of the Department of Sociology in the College of Liberal Arts and Sciences and to the Graduate School and was accepted as partial fulfillment of the requirements for the degree of Doctor of Philosophy.

December 2000

____

Dean, Graduate School

CPSIA information can be obtained
at www.ICGtesting.com
Printed in the USA
BVHW011658100619
550610BV00011B/472/P